Contents

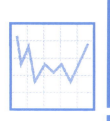

Published as a seperate document:

Volume 2 – Protocol for Assessing Services for People with Severe Mental Illness (Version 2 protocol)
ISBN 0 11 321 922 9

Preface

The Clinical Standards Advisory Group (CSAG) was established in April 1991, under Section 62 of the National Health Service (NHS) and Community Care Act 1990, as an independent source of expert advice to the UK Health Ministers and to the NHS on standards of clinical care for, and access and availability of services to, NHS patients. Remits are set by the UK Health Ministers in discussion with the Group.

The Group's members are nominated by the medical, nursing and dental Royal Colleges and their Faculties, and include the Chairmen of the Standing Medical, Nursing and Midwifery, and Dental Advisory Committees. Its investigations are carried out by members and co-opted experts, supported by research units under contract. Financial support is provided by the UK Health Departments, and the secretariat is based in the Department of Health, Room 409, Wellington House, 133/155 Waterloo Road, London, SE1 8UG.

Sir Gordon Higginson
Chairman, Clinical Standards Advisory Group
February 1995

Clinical Standards Advisory Group:

616.8982.

8640

Schizophrenia. Volume 1

Report of a CSAG Committee
on Schizophrenia: Volume 1

Chaired by Professor Andrew Sims

August 1995

London HMSO

ISBN 0 11 321 929 6

Other titles in this series of CSAG reports are available from HMSO Books and include:

Access to and Availability of Specialist Services
0 11 321 596 7

Coronary Artery Bypass Grafting and Coronary Angioplasty: access to and availability of specialist services
0 11 321 597 5

Childhood Leukaemia: access to and availability of specialist services
0 11 321 598 3

Neonatal Intensive Care: access to and availability of specialist services
011 321 599 1

Cystic Fibrosis: access to and availabilty of specialist services
0 11 321 600 9

Standards of Clinical Care for People with Diabetes
0 11 321 819 2

Back Pain
0 11 321 887 7

Epidemiology Review: the Epidemiology and Cost of Back Pain
0 11 321 889 3

Urgent and Emergency Admissions to Hospital
0 11 321 835 4

Women in Normal Labour
0 11 321 923 7

Dental General Anaesthesia
0 11 321 924 5

Schizophrenia Volume 2
0 11 321 922 9

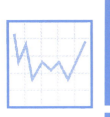

Executive Summary

Up to 1 in 100 people are likely to suffer from schizophrenia at some point in their lifetime. About £1 billion a year is spent on health and personal social services for them.

CSAG was asked by the UK Health Ministers to advise on the standards of clinical care being achieved for people with schizophrenia. CSAG assessed mental health services in eleven NHS Districts and Boards against a study protocol of 156 questions based on current standards of professional good practice. Visiting teams found widely varying achievement of these standards both between provider units and across standards. Interviews with users and carers and with social services confirmed the extent of variation. High standards were being achieved for some aspects of services in all districts. Examples of good practice are identified throughout the report.

Four of the eleven districts approached an overall profile of achievement that CSAG characterised as "good"; for two the profile was, broadly, "poor". The most important single feature distinguishing good from poor was staff morale. CSAG's overall conclusion was that quality of care for those suffering from schizophrenia was in several districts unsatisfactory when assessed against objective standards. Improvement in standards depends primarily on local identification, and then rectification, of specific weaknesses. This will have cost implications where improvements require action beyond better use of present resources.

CSAG's general recommendation is that all mental health services should be appraised locally against the revised CSAG protocol (in Volume 2, ISBN 0 11 321 922 9 available from HMSO); and that, in districts with weaknesses, all those concerned with services for people suffering from severe mental illness, including schizophrenia, should act to improve local levels of care.

Issues to which CSAG believes all mental health services should give attention are

- setting explicit local standards, in consultation with users and carers

- inter-agency working

- multi-professional audit, emphasising clinical diagnosis

- implementing the Care Programme Approach, supported by patient-based registers, and improved resources for areas of particular need

- clinical leadership

Specific recommendations are:

1   The Version 2 protocol should be further developed through wider use by clinicians, managers and commissioners as part of their local audit measures

2   Commissioners should, after consulting users and carers, agree with service providers explicit statements of the standards to be achieved locally, and consider referring in these statements to use of the Version 2 protocol, as developed, as one of the methods of auditing clinical and managerial aspects of the district service.

3   The NHS Executive should, where it has serious concerns about standards and the effectiveness of local audit to identify weaknesses, consider using the Version 2 protocol itself or inviting an independent agency to investigate in more detail.

4   The place of skilled diagnosis within the clinical and social assessment of people with severe mental illness in indicating priority for services should be recognised in contracts, supported and audited.

5   A simple register system should be developed to support the information requirements of the Care Programme Approach, with Supervision Registers and Supervised Discharge as subsets, and to underpin clinical work with high priority groups and clinical audit.

6   The principles of multi-disciplinary and multi-professional audit should be applied in all agencies providing care for designated groups such as the severely mentally ill. This will require harmonisation of methods of data collection by local mental health teams, general practices and social services.

7   CSAG should repeat its district surveys following discussion with districts regarding the visiting teams' assessments of standards and priorities for change.

Chapter 1

Introduction

"It is to the weakest and most unfortunate that society owes most diligent protection and care" (Jean Colombier, 1736-1789)

1.1   In early 1993 there were public and professional concerns about how the care of people with severe mental illness would be affected by the conjunction of three changes: the transfer of care from institutions to the community, which had been gathering momentum over several decades; the NHS Reforms under the NHS and Community Care Act 1990, which were being implemented from 1991; and the community care aspects of that Act, which were to be implemented in full in April 1993. Accordingly the Clinical Standards Advisory Group (CSAG) proposed that it should monitor and assess standards of clinical care for people with schizophrenia as a discrete clinical condition that typified the services for severely mentally ill people.

1.2   In August 1993 the Secretary of State for Health, on behalf of the UK Health Ministers, asked CSAG:

"To advise on standards of clinical care for people with a diagnosis of schizophrenia. You will review existing clinical standards; and report on how these standards are being reflected in NHS contracts and on the extent to which they are being met by health care providers in an illustrative sample of districts and boards. You will specifically investigate the effectiveness of measures in place to audit the standards of clinical care being delivered, including the process of diagnosis and assessment; the use being made of the Care Programme Approach for people with schizophrenia living in the community; and the interface between health authorities and the purchasers and providers of social care in relation to co-operation, co-ordination, and liaison designed to produce a seamless service."

This was announced as part of a Ten Point Plan to reinforce community care for mentally ill people (see Appendix 7).

1.3   CSAG established a Schizophrenia Committee chaired by Professor Andrew Sims and composed of CSAG members and co-opted experts (membership listed at Appendix 5). The Committee asked the Royal College of Psychiatrists' Research Unit to collate existing statements of clinical standards; and then, following a wider invitation to tender, commissioned the Unit to support its members in assessing services in a sample of NHS units against a protocol based on those standards. A programme of visits by members and multi-disciplinary teams (listed at Appendix 6) took place in spring 1994.

1.4   In designing its study the Committee drew upon the experience of the Health Advisory Service, whose Director was co-opted as a member. CSAG also discussed its work with officers of the Audit Commission, which was at that time carrying out a value-for-money audit of mental health services on which it has since reported ("Finding A Place", HMSO 1994). CSAG is grateful to them, to the members of the visiting teams , and to the many people who gave their time during its visits.

1.5   CSAG is a UK body. For simplicity, throughout this report the term "district" is used to include Health Boards in Scotland and Health and Social Service Boards in Northern Ireland, as well as Health Districts in England and Wales; and the term "region" is used to include Scotland, Wales and Northern Ireland as well as the eight Health Regions in England.

Chapter 2

Epidemiology, Treatment and Costs

Clinical background

2.1   Mental illness is a general term used to describe a group of disorders that vary greatly in form and degree of severity. This report is not concerned, for example, with dementia, learning disability, drug or alcohol use, mild neurotic or depressive disorders. The research is focused on schizophrenia because this is the commonest mental disorder associated both with referral to emergency psychiatric services and - as a result of chronic disabilities and the relative young age of onset - because it leads to long-term contact with residential or day facilities or family care. Other severe mental illnesses, such as the severe affective, bipolar (manic-depressive) disorders, present different clinical pictures and require different treatment regimes, but from the point of view of contracting for services many of the problems are similar. It is therefore reasonable, within limits, to use schizophrenia as a proxy for *severe mental illness* more generally.

2.2   Schizophrenia is no different from other illnesses in that it is necessary to understand the nature of the problems experienced by those afflicted in order to be able to provide the most effective help. A brief and non-technical description of the commonest symptoms and the general course of the disorder is included in order to illustrate why services are necessary. There are two main groups, often called 'positive' and 'negative'.

2.3   The *positive symptoms* are prominent in acute attacks and may sometimes continue over longer periods. Afflicted people complain, that their own thoughts, perceptions and intentions are distorted. They may experience their thoughts echoed or commented upon, hear loud and threatening voices that no-one else can hear, and adopt explanations that other people regard as 'crazy'. The experiences, however, are subjectively real, not imaginary. It is not surprising that intense anxiety, depression or excitement often accompany such symptoms or that behaviour may be affected adversely. It is when such experiences and beliefs become distressing, both to themselves and others notably their relatives and friends, and may have serious results if acted upon, that help is necessary.

2.4   Repeated acute attacks present a further liability to someone afflicted by schizophrenia, particularly if preventive help is not rapidly forthcoming and the social environment is characterised by stigma and neglect. Such attacks can be preceded, accompanied and followed by *negative symptoms* that tend to be longer-lasting, such as emotional blunting, slowness of thought and movement, under activity, lack of drive, difficulty with verbal and non-verbal communication, and withdrawal from social contacts. These disabilities tend to be chronic and not responsive to medication.

2.5   The course of schizophrenia therefore depends not only on the particular mix of symptoms and their recurrence and persistence but on the quality of the interpersonal and social environment and of the help available.

The term 'Schizophrenia'

2.6   Using a name is sometimes called 'labelling', with the implication that stigma can be avoided if no name is used. In fact, stigma accrues because of the nature of the manifestations and their effects on behaviour. Publicity is given to a relatively small number of tragic incidents that are clearly linked to the illness, thus giving an impression that all afflicted people are likely to be violent, whereas the vast majority are not. But alternative labels tend to be much more vague and pejorative and do not suggest the hope (many clinicians would say the near-certainty) that schizophrenia will one day be fully understood and means of cure or prevention be found. Meanwhile, there is no implication that using the term clinically means that biomedical factors outweigh the well-known psychosocial factors involved in causation, treatment and care, as will be described below. In fact, attempting to do without the label can mean that priority is not given to the most severe psychiatric disorders that require it. It is clear that such lack of care can lead to relapse, sometimes with serious consequences that may alienate the public (thus indeed giving schizophrenia an adverse image), lead to separation from family and friends, and to self-harm.

The leading charities representing the views of those afflicted and their families use the term in their titles (NSF - National Schizophrenia Fellowship and SANE - Schizophrenia: A National Emergency). Manic-depressive, or Bipolar Disorder, is similarly acknowledged. Until a convincing case is made for another term, 'schizophrenia' should continue to be used.

Statistics and epidemiology

2.7   About one person in a hundred is likely at some time during a lifetime to suffer from the disorder. The frequency of first onset (incidence) is about one in 10,000 population each year. Thus an average general practice with a list size of 2,100 can expect one new patient to present about every four years. At any one time, between 3 and 4 per 1,000 of the general population are experiencing problems associated with schizophrenia; in the whole of the UK, about 150-220,000 people.

2.8   The peak frequency of onset is in the early twenties. Onset is generally about five years earlier in men than in women. Following a first attack there remains a definite vulnerability to recurrence and to the development of long-term disability. However, using combined measures of outcome such as symptom severity, occupation, partnership and degree of dependence, about a quarter recover well within five years. The problems of another two-thirds fluctuate over decades, often with good periods of reasonable functioning. About 10-15 per cent develop severe long-term incapacity. At any one time, therefore, afflicted people are less likely to be employed or living with a partner than people of the same sex or similar age in the general population.

2.9   Standardised mortality rates in schizophrenia are 2.5 times higher than those for the rest of the population; 10-15% of people who develop the disorder eventually commit suicide.

2.10   There is good evidence that schizophrenia is commoner in the centre of large cities and associated with conditions of poverty, poor housing, no housing (30% of those living 'on the streets'), unemployment, and social isolation. Indicators of social deprivation, such as the Jarman index, are positively correlated with admission rates.

Treatment and care

2.11   In the light of these figures, it is perhaps not surprising that schizophrenia accounts for 42.5% of all bed days in mental health specialist care in England. A recent survey of inner London psychiatric hospitals found a 'true bed occupancy' (including beds not occupied because patients were on leave or on supervised discharge programmes) of 130%. Half the patients were admitted compulsorily under a section of the Mental Health Act. Less deprived areas tend to have fewer such problems.

2.12   The basic causes of schizophrenia are not known with any degree of certainty and there are no certain means of primary prevention. There is a genetic contribution in many cases and possibly an increased risk from environmental causes such as exposure to viral infection during the mother's pregnancy. There is also substantial empirical knowledge about the alleviating effects of several kinds of treatment and care. One of these is medication, which is usually effective to a worthwhile degree in controlling the positive symptoms in spite of the liability to produce unwanted side-effects. The recent introduction of medications that promise to help the negative symptoms is still experimental. However, as with all treatments that may have to be continued over a long period of time, it is essential to monitor medication regularly and carefully and to combine with, and if necessary substitute other methods of treatment.

2.13   Much is known about the effects of the psychosocial environment on both positive and negative symptoms in schizophrenia. Too much pressure or stress is likely to exacerbate any tendency towards positive symptoms, while too little encouragement to maintain an optimal level of activity can lead to the negative symptoms getting worse. Achieving a balance requires well-trained multi-disciplinary staff with the knowledge and skills between them to understand and use a range of therapeutic measures, help the self-knowledge of patients, keep an eye on welfare arrangements and physical health and promote the caring efforts of family and friends. Cognitive methods of therapy are of value when distressing symptoms persist. Many sufferers can learn how to control symptoms to some extent, and relatives can learn how to help. The problems of 'living with schizophrenia', like those of living with any other handicapping condition, are not immutable.

2.14   In order to exercise these skills to best effect, a range of treatment settings is required, providing opportunities for continuity of interaction between staff and patients over appropriate periods of time, with an emphasis on preserving the maximum possible autonomy and dignity. Apart from residential accommodation for assessment and care in and following acute emergencies, these include hostels with varied staffing levels (24 hours, 'sleep-in', daytime-only, 'secure' and 'direct access'), group homes, supervised lodgings, and skilled assistance to patients and relatives within their own homes. Occupational and recreational opportunities are equally important and include rehabilitation units, sheltered workshops, day hospitals and centres, and dining and social clubs. The study protocol at Appendix 1 is based on this principle.

Costs

2.15   Residential services are the most costly form of care for the mentally ill. The rundown of large mental hospitals has reduced the numbers of very long-term residents but expenditure has not reduced proportionately. Many hospitals remain open with smaller numbers and it is not clear that closing others has always resulted in the savings being retained for community alternatives. At the same time, the general hospital wards have higher unit costs and special services created to care for people with acute disorders without admission have not proved much cheaper.

2.16   In 1992/3, the total amount spent on the mental health services in England alone was £2.6 billion. This consisted of about £1,780m for in-patient care, £160m for out-patients, £120m for day patients, £250m for community health services and £200m for personal social services. About £1 billion of this is for people with schizophrenia. These figures include neither Family Health Services (eg a net ingredient cost of £17m for anti-psychotic drugs and depot injection), Income Support for independent residential care, nor costs to patients, families and society more generally (which are substantial, though difficult to calculate and often not acknowledged).

2.17 Summary of key facts about schizophrenia

- The main problems for people with schizophrenia include: distressing hallucinations, delusions, depression, anxiety; impaired functioning in activities, thought and communication, all affecting daily living skills; associated behavioural problems; associated interpersonal and social problems.

- The resulting disablement leads to specific needs for help, care, services and sometimes protection.

- Up to 1 in 100 of the population suffers from schizophrenia at some point during a lifetime; the onset is earlier, and the prognosis less favourable, in men. A general practice with a list size of 1,900 will expect to see about 1 new-onset case every 4 years or so; the highest incidence is before 25 years old.

- At any one time, between 3 and 4 per 1,000 of the general population are experiencing problems associated with schizophrenia.

- After a first episode, about one-quarter make a good recovery within 5 years, two thirds will have multiple episodes with some degree of disability between them, and 10-15% will develop severe continuous incapacity.

- Schizophrenia accounts for about 50% of acute admissions to psychiatric wards, 60% of those staying for more than 6 months, and 75% of those in longer-term residential care.

- Of all those on an active list for contact with specialist psychiatric services (other than for dementia or severe learning disability) about half are likely to have schizophrenia.

- Standardised mortality rates in schizophrenia are $2\frac{1}{2}$ times those of the rest of the population; 45% with long-term conditions also have physical illnesses, particularly cardiovascular and respiratory.

- 15% of those with long-term schizophrenia die from suicide.

- People with schizophrenia are often socially isolated and disadvantaged.

- There are more people with schizophrenia in deprived and isolated areas of the country, particularly inner cities.

- One-third of people sleeping rough have schizophrenia.

- Half of those referred for psychiatric report from the magistrates' courts in inner London had suffered from schizophrenia. Only one quarter of those referred had a settled address.

- Family members make a substantial, unpaid, contribution to the care of people with long-term disablement associated with schizophrenia.

Chapter 3

Methods

Introduction

3.1   CSAG's overall method collated existing standards and prepared a protocol of questions to assess the extent to which clinical services were meeting those standards. It then asked those questions in visits to a sample of NHS districts, collected other data and documents and analysed this information.

Standards

3.2   In order to assess the standards of clinical care being achieved in a sample of Districts, CSAG's practice in all its studies is first to identify, or help articulate, such standards and guidelines as command a professional consensus. Its intention in doing so is to inform its inquiries, not to set new standards. As with clinical audit, CSAG aims to help the NHS improve practice, and does not expect ideal standards to be universally applied.

3.3   CSAG's Schizophrenia Committee identified no single clear statement of clinical standards, either for the clinical care that people with schizophrenia should receive or for the services that should be provided. At CSAG's request, the Royal College of Psychiatrists' Research Unit convened a multidisciplinary panel to search the literature and prepare a detailed statement of existing guidelines and standards.

The protocol

3.4   The Unit then drafted questions concerning the provision of services based on those standards (the "study protocol", see Appendix 1). In view of the practical difficulties in defining and measuring clinical care, the protocol concentrates on describing factors to be taken into account during the purchasing process and on what providers could be expected to deliver; and on providing methods of rating that allow assessment of each District for each item. CSAG did not construct clinical guidelines for specific aspects of clinical care, for example detailed medication regimes, since these could have been audited only by assessing their use for individual patients. That would not have been possible in this kind of survey, and should be the subject of local audit by professional peer review - questions about which were included in the protocol.

3.5   In order to help identify questions pertinent to the - then relatively new - purchasing process, CSAG commissioned the University of Birmingham to analyse 25% of purchaser-provider contracts for mental illness in England for 1992/93. This found that the gap between best and worst practice in purchasing was considerable, and contract documentation in a few authorities amounted to little more than a memo for regulating the transfer of funds. The majority of purchasers were committed to the treatment of severe mental illness on a multi-agency (61%) and multi-disciplinary (59%) basis, in the community rather than hospital wherever practicable (54%); less than a quarter (22%) proposed to develop the home treatment model of acute care. Almost all (95%) purchasers included lists of quality standards in their contract documentation, of which the most common were that patients (83%) and their carers (71%) should be informed about the patient's illness and legal rights, and that the Care Programme Approach (77%) and clinical audit procedures (66%) be implemented. Few purchasers (15%) specified health gain targets, reflecting the unavailability of routinely-collected outcome information in mental health services. Part 1 of the CSAG study protocol, on purchaser-provider interactions, was then developed in collaboration with Dr Cumella of the University of Birmingham and Dr Williams of the Health Advisory Service (who subsequently reviewed all contracts for 1993/94, a report on which is being prepared by the Health Advisory Service).

3.6   All items in the protocol are in the form either of positive statements that are relatively simple to affirm or deny, with supporting evidence, or of measures that can be quantified more precisely, on the assumption that such information should normally be available to purchasers and providers. Quantifications are simplified as ratings on scales showing the extent of achievement or the rapidity with which the service can be made available to an individual. Both types of item can be checked on a list, so that progress could in future be measured. CSAG required evidence to show that positive answers were justified and noted "good practice" believed to have contributed to such answers. CSAG aimed to provide a wide range of measures against which a profile of achievement could be built up for each District, recognising that this will vary by District and over time, and look for overall achievement rather than a "pass" or "fail" against pre-set minimum acceptable levels for individual measures. Each District's profile will have its own implications for local priorities in developing services.

3.7   The draft protocol, and an outline of CSAG's overall method, were considered at a national CSAG conference in March 1994, attended by representatives of user and carer organisations, social services, and professional bodies. The conference broadly agreed the protocol but suggested adding visits to social services departments and users and carers to the arrangements for visits to health districts. This was subsequently agreed by CSAG with the Association of Directors of Social Services.

3.8   The protocol was also refined during two informal pilot visits. It will be further developed to reflect experience gained during the project and the amended version will be available as Volume 2 to this report. Suggestions made by members of the visiting teams for consideration when revising the protocol are at Appendix 3. It should be further amended as clinical guidelines and/or outcome measures become available and as information systems for both services and clinical quality improve; and should take account of the "Good Practice Statement on Services for People Affected By Schizophrenia" being prepared by Scottish Office CRAG/SCOTMEG Working Group.

3.9   CSAG could not in the time available repeat its visits, but recognises that the protocol is best used within an audit cycle. Revisiting at intervals, and post-visit discussion of findings, would be included in any longer-term study methodology, which would help Districts to gradually improve their all-round audit profile.

Visiting teams

3.10 Each team was made up of three or four members from different professions including members of CSAG's Schizophrenia Committee and experts selected with the aid of the appropriate professional bodies and supported by a senior member of the research team. The team for each visit included a consultant psychiatrist and a mental health nurse; the remaining members alternated between psychology, social work and occupational therapy. Members of the teams are listed in Appendix 6.

3.11   Team members and the research unit took part in a training course in March 1994 organised by the Health Advisory Service and based on a model they had recently developed for training HAS visitors. The two day course, at the Civil Service College, included details of CSAG's audit approach, protocol and organisation; purchasing issues; and interview techniques and role playing for the interviews that the teams would carry out on their district visits.

Procedure for visits

3.12   About four weeks before the main visit a researcher met, separately, nominated liaison officers from the Health Authority and the Trust or directly managed provider unit to collect information and documents and to devise a provisional timetable of meetings and visits to facilities.

3.13   The main visits by the multidisciplinary team lasted two days. On the first morning the team met representatives of the purchasing authority, usually from Public Health, to work through Part 1 of the (Version 1) protocol on the purchaser-provider interaction. On the first afternoon the team met senior managers and clinicians of the main provider unit and worked through Part 2 on the provision of services. The providers rated themselves on each item; team members concurrently made their own ratings and asked for information and clarification of each item the provider rated. The team then met to discuss the information gathered, to re-rate the items jointly and to highlight specific issues for investigation the following day.

3.14   The second day of the visit was spent at local NHS facilities. Often the team split into 2 or 3 groups. As far as possible the teams visited acute admission wards, intensive care/secure wards, long stay/rehabilitation wards, day hospital and centres, occupational therapy departments, Community Psychiatric Nurse or Community Mental Health Team bases, and hostel/residential care homes. The team met again at the end of the day to pool information, make their final ratings and record their impressions.

3.15   Information from social service departments and user/carer organisations concerning provision of specialist mental health care was collected after the completion of the team visits. A member of the research team contacted and visited the relevant organisations in each district for their views on the range and quality of services provided by the NHS for people with schizophrenia.

3.16   It was not possible in the time available to visit GP practices, although several GPs attended meetings in provider units or at facilities. CSAG was also mindful of its present statutory limitation, under Section 62(7) of the NHS & Community Care Act 1990, to Hospital and Community Health Services: CSAG can consider links with Family Health Services and with Personal Social Services, but not standards within those services. (The Health Authorities Bill currently before Parliament proposes amending Section 62(7) so that CSAG could in future advise on all services for which the new Health Authorities will be responsible, including Family Health Services.) At the time of designing the study few GPs in most Districts visited were Fund Holders, and Fund Holding had only recently been extended to include the purchasing of community (not in-patient) mental health services (see chapter 3.25 below). Any similar study now would need to interview Fund Holders as well as DHA purchasers.

3.17   The District visits took place between April and June 1994. Visits to user and carer representatives and to social services departments continued into the autumn.

Selection of districts

3.18 CSAG's intention was to select an illustrative sample of mental health services throughout the UK, allowing for the practical constraint of completing the work in a limited period. The selection therefore took account of:

a   **Country: one district in each of Scotland, Wales and Northern Ireland and in the eight new Regions in England.**

b   **Deprivation (according to Jarman index or similar measure).**

c   **Urban and rural environments.**

d   **Teaching and non-teaching districts.**

e   **Proximity to, or recent closure of, a psychiatric hospital.**

3.19 It is a principle of CSAG that units in the NHS selected for inclusion in the sample studied are assured that they will be anonymised in CSAG's reports to Ministers; and that staff are assured that information provided by them is in confidence. CSAG's assessments of units are reported to those units, with due protection for individual sources of information as appropriate. In the Tables, districts are identified only by the letters A–K.

Data collection

3.20 Quantitative data were requested from purchaser and provider organisations. Data request forms were completed by clinical liaison officers in liaison with Trust information departments and the research unit. Many districts reported that they were unable to produce reliable figures for many of the items requested, and so had to give estimates. Further data were collected from central sources and from local district public health departments (suicide rates, unemployment rates etc.). Volumes and health service indicators were too patchy or unreliable to be used for comparative purposes. Useful data collected from central and local public health sources included population size, unemployment rates, percentage of ethnic minorities, Jarman Underprivileged Area 8-item (UPA8) scores and rankings, standard mortality ratios, and suicide rates. These are anonymised and listed in Table 1.

3.21 A crude comparison between the mean Jarman score for the one Welsh and eight English districts selected for this study (+10.3) and that for districts at the mid-point of the national Jarman ranking (-2.81, range -29.2 to +63.4) shows the study mean to be a little on the deprived side of the national figure. In view of the small sample such comparisons must be interpreted very cautiously.

Analysis of protocol data

3.22 The protocol (Appendix 1) contains 156 ratable items: 44 covering purchaser topics; and 112 provider topics. The purchaser items are all rated Yes or No. Several types of rating are used for the provider items. The methods of rating are described in Appendix 2.

3.23 The first stage in the analysis was to devise a method for summarising the large amount of information collected. Following the two pilot assessments of districts not included in the main study a list of key points was prepared by the research unit, seven for purchasers and eleven for providers, based on the protocol ratings and the teams' overall impressions of the range and quality of services. These key points are outlined in Tables 2 and 3.

Table 1. Socio-economic characteristics

	District A	District B	District C	District D	District E	District F	District G	District H	District I	District J	District K
Population Size	Large	Small	Medium	Medium	Large	Small	Medium	Small	Large	Medium	Medium
Unemployment Rate	Medium	High	High	High	High	Medium	High	Low	Medium	High	Low
Ethnic Minority	Low	Low	Low	Medium	Medium	Low	High	Medium	Medium	High	Medium
Deprivation (from Jarman)	Low	Medium	Low	Medium	Medium	Medium	High	Low	Medium	Medium	Medium
Standardised Mortality Rate	Low	High	Low	Low	High	Low	Low	Low	Low	High	High
Large Psychiatric Hospital	Closing	None	Yes	None	Closing	Yes	None	None	Yes	None	None
Rural/Urban	Rural & Urban	Urban, Industrial	Rural & Urban	Urban, Industrial	Urban, industrial & inner city	Urban, industrial	Urban, industrial & inner city	Rural & urban	Rural & urban	Urban, industrial	Urban, industrial & inner city
Suicide Rate	High	Low	Low	High	Medium	Low	High	Medium	Medium	Medium	Low

Notes

Population Size: Small<200,000; Medium 200,000-399,999; Large>400,000 (Mean population of Districts A–K=300,000)

Unemployment Rate: Low<6%; Medium 6-12%; High>12% (UK Unemployment Rate 1991=8.7%)

Ethnic Minority: Low<1%; Medium 1-10%; High>10% (UK Ethnic Minority 1991=5.8%, Mean ethnic minority of Districts A–K=6.6%)

Deprivation (Jarman Index): Low<1; Medium 1-40; High>40 (Two mid-ranked district scores=-2.81, Airedale & North East Essex)

Standardised Morality Ratio: Low<100; High>100 (UK standard=100)

Suicide Rate:Low<8%; Medium 8-12%; High>12% (Mean Suicide Rate of Districts A–K=9.3%)

14

Table 2. Key points for assessing purchasers

1   **Strategic Plan** - the district has carried out strategy development in conjunction with other key stakeholders to ensure a unified approach

2   **Review and updating of strategic plan** - procedure and timetable for review and update of strategic plan

3   **Population-based needs assessment** - methodology and procedure for population-based needs assessment

4   **Service specification** - a detailed specification including statements of services for people with severe mental illness.

5   **Explicit targets and quality standards** - which should be set out in the service specification or contract

6   **Regular contract monitoring meetings** - formal systems set in place for purchasers and providers to meet on a regular basis

7   **Purchasers ensure that providers implement and monitor statutory guidelines** - for CPA, supervision registers, medical/clinical audit, Mental Health Act Code of Practice etc

Table 3. Key points for assessing providers

1   **Business Plan** - that there is a business plan.

2   **Service directory** - that there is a service directory.

3   **Involvement of clinical staff in contracting** - that there are effective mechanisms for clinicians' views to be communicated directly to the purchasers.

4   **Care Programme Approach** - that there is a policy and register for the CPA.

5   **Section 117 of the Mental Health Act** - that there is some form of register and monitoring of individuals subject to the requirements of section 117.

6   **Users and Carers actively involved in services** - local organisations should be actively involved in the planning process and the monitoring of quality.

7   **Advocacy supported and facilitated** - advocacy schemes or workers, either directly funded or from user groups.

8   **Quality of residential accommodation** - the quality of both the physical and social environment.

9   **Full range of accessible services** - that there is full range of services accessible to those with severe mental illness.

10 **Specialist practitioners/teams for schizophrenia or severe mental illness.**

11 **Audit** - active and routine audits are effective in improving the quality of clinical practices and services.

12 **Social Services** - social services' views of local NHS services for those with schizophrenia.

13 **Users and Carers** - users' and carers' views of local NHS services for those with schizophrenia.

3.24 A member of the research team took part in all the main visits and, immediately following each one, made a summary profile of how far each district had met the key criteria. Each key point was rated on a scale from 0 (absent), through 1 (poor), 2 (moderate) and 3 (good), to 4 (excellent). Subsequently, contacts were made with local social services departments and local user and carer groups. Ratings of their comments upon specialist health services added two further key points to the provider list, making 13 in all. Thus a profile of 20 key points was constructed that could be used to assess the extent to which districts had met the standards laid down in the Protocol.

Purchasing and providing services

3.25 The Purchasing and Providing functions in the NHS were formally separated in April 1991 as part of the implementation of the NHS and Community Care Act 1990. At that time the purchasers of health care for mentally ill people were almost exclusively District Health Authorities (DHAs), with Regional Health Authorities responsible for purchasing some highly specialised services. GP fundholding (GPFH) practices could purchase only out-patient mental health services and, from April 1993, community mental health services.

3.26 In this study the specific purchasing role of GPFHs was not explored in detail; the proportion of the local population covered by GPFHs in our sample of Districts was small in all but one, affluent, rural area. The visiting teams did not meet GPFHs formally during the visits. Information from a number of providers indicated that, in some districts, the impact of fundholding on care for people with severe mental illness, at both primary and secondary care levels, is already significant, but this would require further study before it could be commented on with authority.

3.27 The terms 'Purchaser' and 'Purchasing' are used throughout this section (and in the Protocol) to describe a range of functions including planning, contracting, needs assessment, financial and performance monitoring. The term 'Commissioning' is increasingly used as an umbrella term for these functions.

3.28 Providers of health care were principally NHS Trusts and some units which had not yet sought or achieved Trust status. These latter are referred to as Directly Managed Units (DMUs), since they remained under the managerial oversight of the DHA. In the CSAG visits, all but two of the NHS provider units had become Trusts.

3.29 The essential feature of this functional separation is that since 1991 it is for DHAs to determine the health care needs of their resident population and, through the process of agreeing service contracts, to ensure that services are commissioned to meet these needs, within the constraints of a fixed financial allocation.

3.30 A review of the standards of care provided for people with schizophrenia, and severe mental illness more generally, must include information about the current arrangements for purchasing mental health services; and must consider, as far as practicable, the arrangements for, and quality of, the interactions between purchasers and providers.

3.31 In all visits CSAG met senior members of the DHA purchasing team. Some CSAG visiting teams reported that they felt at a disadvantage in meeting purchasers if their team did not include a member with experience in purchasing. It is possible that this factor might have influenced the teams' ability to question or challenge responses from the purchasers. Nevertheless, the procedure for information collection emphasised the systematic use of the Protocol together with the background documentation and the information from the 'scouting' visits.

Chapter 4 | Results

District ratings on key points

4.1   The results of our analysis of protocol data are presented as summary ratings for each key point in Tables 4 and 5 for purchasers and providers respectively (scores for all provider items in the protocol are in Table 7 at Appendix 2).

4.2   As a first approximation to a classification of districts according to the quality of purchasing and providing services for the severely mentally ill, their ratings on key points were summed to provide a subtotal for purchasers per district (7 items, range 0-28), a subtotal for providers and others (13 items, range 0-52), and a total score (20 items, range 0-80). These are shown in Table 6.

Table 4. Summary ratings for purchaser

	District A	District B	District C	District D	District E	District F	District G	District H	District I	District J	District K
Strategic plan	3	4	2	3	3	2	1	0	2	1	1
Review and updating of strategic plan	3	3	2	3	3	2	2	2	4	1	2
Population based needs assessment	2	3	2	2	3	2	2	1	3	1	1
Service specification	3	3	2	3	2	2	1	2	1	1	1
Explicit targets & quality standards	2	3	3	2	3	1	1	1	0	1	1
Regular contract meetings with providers	2	2	3	2	2	2	2	2	1	1	1
Explicit references to best practice guidelines	3	3	2	3	2	2	2	2	2	1	1
Total	**18**	**21**	**16**	**18**	**18**	**13**	**11**	**10**	**13**	**7**	**8**

Rating:

0 nil, no evidence; 1 minimal/poor; 2 some/moderate; 3 good; 4 excellent.

18

Table 5. Summary ratings for providers

	District A	District B	District C	District D	District E	District F	District G	District H	District I	District J	District K
Business plan	3	3	2	2	2	3	0	1	1	0	1
Service directory	2	3	0	4	1	0	2	3	0	0	0
Involvement of clinical staff in contracting	2	3	3	2	1	1	2	1	1	0	1
Care Programme Approach	2	3	3	1	2	2	3	2	1	1	1
Section 117 of Mental Health Act	3	2	2	3	0	2	2	3	3	1	1
Users & carers are actively involved in services	3	3	3	3	2	2	2	0	2	2	0
Advocacy is supported and facilitated	2	2	3	3	2	3	3	0	1	2	0
Quality of residential accommodation	4	2	2	1	2	2	1	2	2	3	1
Full range of accessible services	4	2	4	2	2	2	2	3	3	1	1
Specialist practitioners/ teams for SCZ/SMI	2	2	4	3	3	4	1	2	0	0	0
Audit	3	2	3	3	2	2	2	2	1	0	1
Social services	4	3	3	3	2	2	2	1	2	1	2
Users & carers	3	2	2	1	2	2	1	3	2	1	1
Total	**37**	**32**	**34**	**31**	**23**	**27**	**23**	**23**	**19**	**12**	**10**

Rating:
0 nil, no evidence; 1 minimal/poor; 2 some/moderate; 3 good; 4 excellent.

19

Table 6. Scores by district

District	Purchaser	Provider	Total
A	18	37	55
B	21	32	53
C	16	34	50
D	18	31	49
E	18	23	41
F	13	27	40
G	11	23	34
H	10	23	33
I	13	19	32
J	7	12	19
K	8	10	18
Total	**153**	**271**	**424**

4.3   Average scores for the 7 purchaser key points (21.9 i.e. 153 divided by 7) and for the 13 provider key points (20.9 i.e. 271 divided by 13) are virtually identical; and the ranking for purchasers and providers would be closely similar (rho = 0.78, p < 0.01). Ranking by the number of items rated good or excellent would give a similar picture. We therefore considered the overall total scores as a means of grouping districts on their performance for purposes of further description and comment.

4.4   In Table 6 it is clear that there is a large gap between the bottom two and the other nine, the scores of which are approximately continuous. Inspecting the individual scores in tables 4 and 5 suggests a cut between the top four and a middle five.

4.5   The top group of four districts has an overall mean score of 2.59 per item, so that they do not quite attain an overall 'good' rating. The middle group's mean item score is 1.80 and that of the lower group is 0.93. This three-way split has been used in Figure 1, which summarises the difference between the key item profiles of top, middle and lower districts. There is very little overlap between the three groups.

4.6   We compared the 'top' four districts with the 'middle' five and the 'lower' two in order to consider difficult questions such as 'what factors make for relatively higher standards in a district?' and 'what kind of help is needed to improve lower standards?'. Our conclusions on their comparative characteristics are at 7.3-15.

4.7   We compared scores with the sociodemographic indices in Table 1, of which five could be used as possible indicators of relative need for services. Because the number of districts is small and in some cases data are missing, it is not possible to make firm estimates. Also, because of the need to preserve anonymity the exact scores cannot be given. On <u>deprivation,</u> the Jarman UPA8 scores for eight districts are sufficiently varied to make a rank correlation feasible. However the correlation is not significant (rho=0.08). The rank correlation for <u>unemployment rates</u> (n=10) is also negligible (-0.13). Two districts have relatively high proportions (18.3% and 18.6%) of <u>ethnic minorities</u> (the other districts all have proportions of 5% or less); these two districts are ranked seventh and tenth on total score. There is little variation between districts in <u>Standardised Mortality Rates</u> or <u>suicide rates</u>. We also noted the rank correlation between the percentage of the local population registered with GP fundholders in eight districts and total score, and this is small but significant (0.31).

20

Figure 1. Groupings of districts

Purchasers (7 Items)

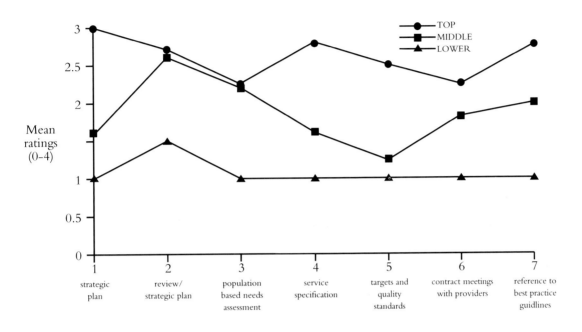

* Top: Districts A-D
  Middle: Districts E-I
  Lower: Districts J-K

Providers (13 items)

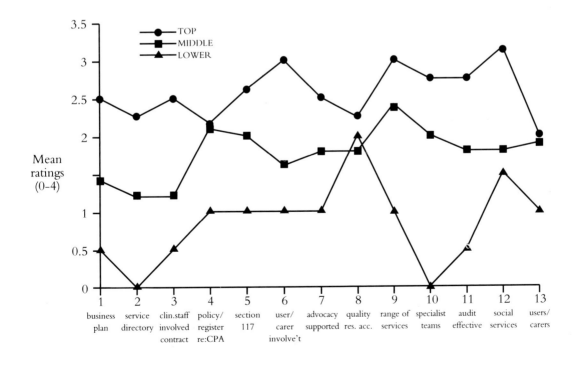

21

Key Purchasing Issues

4.8 Results on purchaser items on the protocol are presented below under the headings of strategic plans, service specifications, contracts, and purchaser-provider interaction. Each group starts with a list of the relevant items from either Part 1 (purchaser items) or Part 2 (provider items) of the Version 1 protocol in Appendix 1, and ends with examples of observed good practice.

Strategic plan for mental health services

Purchaser items in protocol: 1,2,3,4,5,6

4.9 Not all of the Districts had produced a strategic plan document, nor had some begun to devise one. Only one District had produced a well developed plan which was used, effectively, to guide the purchasing plan and contract negotiations, and which was also linked closely to the Community Care Plan. Other Districts appeared to have a strategic approach to purchasing without a specific document to define and describe this strategy. Few strategic plan documents specified proposals for meeting the needs of people with schizophrenia or severe mental illness.

> **One purchaser had developed a strategic plan based on local needs assessment and involvement of interested parties. This document specifically targeted the needs of those with severe mental illness and was used to inform the contracting process. It also had a timetable for review.**

A service specification

Purchaser items in protocol: 7,8,9,10

4.10 The service specification is used to set out, inter alia, details of the three cornerstones of purchasing: costs, volumes; and quality standards. These details are included, or referred to, in the service contract. Ideally the service specification will include a requirement of the provider to implement and observe statutory and national policy directives and nationally agreed targets or good practice protocols.

4.11 Few purchasers developed their service specifications from a 'bottom up' approach, using local information to fine-tune the nationwide information based on policy directives. One purchasing team commented that they were contracting with a third wave Trust provider (i.e. April 1993) and therefore had had insufficient time to develop expertise in preparing contract documentation. They had agreed that a senior manager in the Trust should write the service specification, which had been accepted, without alteration, by the purchasing team.

4.12 Most purchasers said that sound local information about mental health needs was simply not available. As a result many specifications were expressed in a very general way, including, for example, performance or quality standards which were developed in other service areas.

> **In one district, the purchaser's Director of Quality, was working very closely with the provider managers and clinicians to agree relevant and measurable service quality standards for inclusion in planned service specifications; these included targets derived from Health of the Nation.**

Service contracts

Purchaser items in protocol: 13-44(incl.)

4.13   In virtually all cases, there was a simple block contract with straightforward contract currencies such as occupied bed days, finished consultant episodes (FCEs), number of out-patient attendances etc. Many purchasers wanted more sophisticated contracts, including information about health gain and/or outcomes, however local information systems could not support this. As to contract monitoring, regular meetings took place between most purchasers and providers. Some purchasers commented that these tended to focus on contract planning rather than monitoring because specific information was not available to allow effective monitoring against targets.

Interaction between purchasers and providers

4.14   The 'quality' of the relationship was judged informally by comments made to the visiting teams, and more objectively by considering the frequency of joint meetings, the involvement of the clinicians in the contracting process, providers' knowledge and accessibility to purchaser managers. Relationships appeared to range from collaborative partnerships to those characterised by mutual suspicion and hostility. There were some clear differences across the districts in the degree to which some purchasers adopted a 'hands off' commissioning role, whilst others seemed reluctant to let go of familiar line management roles characteristic of pre-1991 arrangements. An example of these different outlooks was seen within one purchasing team: a senior officer stated that they (the purchaser) should not involve themselves in telling clinicians how to do things; another, in the same meeting, expressed the view that they should be involved in monitoring how 'our' (sic) psychiatrists and 'our' community mental health teams deliver services.

4.15   The question of what characterises a 'good' service, in comparison to a moderate or poor one, is discussed in Chapter 8. One factor however, which emerges from the informal comments made to the visiting teams, and from the analysis of scores in Tables 2 and 3, is that 'good' purchasers and 'good' providers tended to be found together.

4.16   About a quarter of the purchasers involved in this study had made impressive efforts to develop good strategic plans on which to base their purchasing decisions. Most others, though not all, had plans to produce good quality strategic documentation, citing lack of expertise in the purchaser team as the commonest reason for lack of progress.

4.17   There was evidence of some confusion in interpreting government policy. At least one purchasing group asserted that they were not required to agree service contracts until their main provider had achieved Trust status in April 1994. Another team appeared to be divided as to the degree to which there should be a "split" between purchaser and provider.

4.18   All purchasers commented on what they saw as a shortage of good quality, relevant information available locally to inform planning, purchasing and monitoring functions.

4.19   Those districts which, in this study, appeared to function best were those where purchasers had a clear strategy in place for purchasing high quality mental health services. They were relatively clear about their role and were able to communicate and share their plans with their providers and with other stakeholders. There was evidence of effective collaboration between health and local authorities resulting in a plan that specified a comprehensive and complementary network of services designed to suit local circumstances.

Key Provider Issues

4.20 The relevant protocol item numbers are listed in a box at the head of each section. Tables showing the ratings for each district and describing the several different methods of rating used are in Table 7 at Appendix 2. Examples of good practice are recorded in a box at the end of each section. 'Good practice' often means achieving good or excellent performance against the standard, but we have tried to find useful illustrations. Some further information about these examples may be obtained by written request from the College Research Unit.

Multidisciplinary team (MDT) review

Purchaser items in protocol: 77

4.21 Regular multidisciplinary team review was an established process in six of the eleven districts, the frequency of reviews varying from 3-monthly to yearly. In four of the six districts, procedures only partially met the standard. For example, in one district regular reviews were undertaken only by consultants. In another, full multidisciplinary team review was confined to those on the Care Programme Approach (CPA) (which at that time had not been implemented for all patients). One district only fully reviewed inpatients. Community Psychiatric Nurses (CPNs) alone were responsible for monitoring patients in the community. Another district only carried out full reviews for inpatients and rehabilitation patients. Five districts did not meet the standard. Two had no policy for multidisciplinary review at all, although some reviews occurred.

> **Several providers included multidisciplinary team review in their Care Programme Approach or team policies. One specified a maximum interval of 12 months (i.e for stable patients); another specified 6 monthly reviews for all patients subject to the Care Programme Approach.**

Assessment of physical health

Purchaser items in protocol: 78

4.22 The policy and practice of monitoring the physical ill health of patients in contact with specialist services varied but were generally unsatisfactory. In two districts monitoring was not undertaken at all. Three districts adopted a policy that physical ill-health was the responsibility of the GP; in one of these the Community Mental Health Team (CMHT) ensured that patients were registered, but did not check that monitoring occurred. In two districts, there was full assessment of physical health only on admission to hospital. In two districts, junior medical staff carried out regular assessments for long stay inpatients. In one, medical staff provided such assessments for all patients.

> **In one district all patients receiving depot neuroleptic medication received a regular physical examination.**

Medication

Purchaser items in protocol: 79,80

4.23 Some monitoring of medication was undertaken in all districts. In four districts, the process was

24

thorough - in some cases with regular support from pharmacists. In three other districts reviews were undertaken but not guided by a systematic policy covering all sites. For example, in one site it would be undertaken by Community Mental Health Team staff, in others by CPNs or depot clinic nurses. In four districts the standard was not sufficiently met; e.g. only those on depot medication received a thorough review by medical and nursing staff. In one of these districts, review was limited to people attending the out patient department. It appeared that no patients were being denied access to drugs like Clozapine, although there were explicit budgetary limits in most districts.

In two sites regular monitoring and review were undertaken by consultant or senior restistrar.

Specific psychological interventions

Purchaser items in protocol: 81,82,83

4.24 The availability of cognitive/behavioural/family approaches was limited in all districts. In two districts these methods were effectively absent. Limited availability is partly due to a lack of trained staff, partly due to geographical and/or organisational factors (different resource allocation to different sectors), and in some cases due to trained staff failing to target the severely mentally ill. The district with the best developed resources gave a service to those suffering acute relapses but people with longer-term disabilities were excluded.

In one district two staff were employed with special expertise in family intervention methods. In order to maximise the benefits of their expertise, they provided support and training to members of the community mental health teams.

One district provided an outstanding service aimed at early intervention in acute illness or relapse designed specifically to avoid admission to hospital.

Continuity of care and the Care Programme Approach (CPA)

Purchaser items in protocol: 9,18,66,67,71,72,73

4.25 The Care Programme Approach (CPA), introduced in England in April 1991 and in Scotland in June 1992, was acknowledged in all districts to enshrine principles of good practice. There was, however, lack of clarity about implementation, which was often poorly co-ordinated and integrated. Many clinicians did not know the procedures involved, either on the ward before discharge or in the community, and this led in turn to complaints that the CPA is cumbersome to apply. Users had little or no understanding of the implications of the CPA and many had never heard of it. Although purchasers knew if the CPA had been implemented in some degree by provider managers, they did not know whether clinicians of all relevant professions understood its implications and were implementing it fully. A written policy, and declared observance of CPA requirements are insufficient to guarantee that the CPA has been fully and properly implemented, and the standards need to be more tightly formulated.

4.26 These difficulties are best tackled through clinical audit and other quality assurance procedures. There is however a clear message to both purchasers and providers that it is essential to be able to demonstrate that CPA is being used, at the very minimum, for patients with severe and/or enduring mental illness. It is insufficient, in contracting, only to require that a policy and procedure for CPA are in place.

4.27 During the time of the visits (April-June 1994), Supervision Registers had not been implemented but in some Districts plans for their use were well advanced. Although many clinicians saw the value of a means of maintaining contact with the most disturbed severely mentally ill in the community, some expressed concerns about confidentiality, practical arrangements, and lack of resources to undertake the necessary work.

One service had good information to support their use of CPA (not computerised) and were able to readily provide useful data to the visiting team, eg. that 90% of key workers were CPNs, the rest social workers.

One service had suffered for several years from an unclear policy and had taken a decision to abandon and start again. A new policy has been developed with broad consultation and agreement to support it. This revised policy and procedure were about to be implemented throughout the trust at the time CSAG visited.

Several districts, including one in a deprived inner city location, had established close and effective links with a number of user and carer groups.

Although the teams found no examples of well-developed computer based record systems, there were examples in two databases of extremely good systems to support the Mental Health Act and Care Programme Approach.

Mental health nursing in the community

Provider items in protocol: 75,76

4.28 Community Psychiatric Nurses (CPNs) - recently redesignated Mental Health Nurses in the Community - have a key role to play in ensuring that people with schizophrenia or other severe mental illness receive the appropriate treatment and care throughout the course of their illness. There was little systematic assessment of mental health nurses' training needs in psychological/family interventions, case management approaches (including assertive outreach), and the assessment of the side effects of medication. Regular clinical supervision, which could guide experience in appropriate targeting of services, coping with workload, and minimising level of stress, was uncommon. Difficult communication between acute inpatient units and community-based teams, within the CPN service itself and between CPNs and psychiatrists, amplified these problems. In some districts, CPNs were unhappy about the stigmatising effects of 'labelling' and did not wish to use the term 'schizophrenia'. This led, on occasion, to a lack of co-ordination between the professions and deployment of their time away from the care of the severely mentally ill. In some districts, CPNs felt uncertainty about their future role and job security.

One trust had a clear policy that CPNs would prioritise the needs of the most severely mentally ill (a re-structuring to provide two sectorised CMHTs was about to take place at the time of the CSAG visit; this prioritisation was to be continued by the newly-formed teams).

Primary care liaison.

Provider items in protocol: 4,5,6,7

4.29 Performance in this area was unsatisfactory. Only four districts provided directories for primary care teams and these were not always comprehensive or easy to access. The mean rating on the other three items was little better than poor. Since general practices were not included in the itinerary of visits, the views recorded here are only of clinicians in the specialist services. Clinicians of all health professions in several districts were concerned about the effects that GP fundholding was beginning to have on practice. Worries were repeatedly expressed (particularly in the district with the highest proportion of fundholding practices) about a possible drift from the priority previously given to the severely mentally ill.

> **One Trust employed a GP Liaison Officer (although this persons role was not confined to mental health).**

Rehabilitation

Provider items in protocol: 54,55,56,57,58,59

4.30 In this area, one district was rated as excellent, four had good ratings on all six items and all districts were at least at a moderate level. Nevertheless, problems of organisation not assessed by these ratings were mentioned in many districts. In some districts there was confusion and a lack of communication between the acute and the longer-term services. For example, in one district a person suffering from schizophrenia had been continuously an inpatient on an acute ward for seven years, despite acceptable rehabilitation services available locally in the community. More specialist rehabilitation services concentrating on secondary prevention in the community might reduce readmission rates among people already known to the service. In several well-equipped and managed districts there was an appropriate level of surveillance and good co-ordination with other agencies. However, in others, there was a lack of internal co-ordination of services. In one rehabilitation service sited in the community, intended for severely mentally ill people, there were no patients suffering from schizophrenia and no alternative day-care was provided in the locality. A further problem mentioned was a lack of appropriately trained staff resulting in a lack of clarity of purpose for the service.

> **An excellent day hospital in an inner city location provides a wide range of activities for people with chronic and debilitating illness despite a modest level of funding.**

Care for those not in touch with services

Provider items in protocol: 52,97,98

4.31 Visiting teams inquired about people with schizophrenia who were homeless or roofless. Five districts had special arrangements but nowhere was it possible to estimate levels of unmet need. The problems raised in section 4.26/28 on continuity of care are relevant to that aspect of homelessness that is due to patients dropping out from care. Clinicians and managers pointed out that commissioning agencies have to ensure that services are purchased to meet the health care needs of the local "resident" population, including homeless people but that many untreated people with severe mental illness are not 'local' and may not be registered with general practitioners. There was usually no specific strategy for making contact with people with untreated schizophrenia in the community, and often no protocol for those who stop attending a mental health facility, unless they are receiving depot injections. Six districts had an arrangement for diversion of mentally ill offenders from court and three could use a bail hostel.

Ethnicity

Provider items in protocol: 84,85,86,87,88

4.32   Three districts had tiny ethnic minorities (<1%), five had proportions of 5% or less and one had 7%. Two had nearly 20%; in one of these there was an established 'black and minority' mental health strategy group and a good awareness of cultural/ethnic factors. Three districts had some links with local community organisations but had yet to develop formal mechanisms or special arrangements for health service managers or operational staff to consult with these groups. One district with several different minority groups said that the communities were 'too varied' to merit a co-ordinated response, whilst another found it difficult to establish contacts with a predominantly Asian population. One district with a very small minority had regular meetings with a local race forum and was providing training for the staff in ethnic issues.

4.33   All districts had some form of access to translators for patients from ethnic communities. The three districts with the largest ethnic groups had good access to interpreting services, but the fourth largest found it difficult to get interpreters for non-English speaking patients because of their poor links with community groups. Districts with smaller ethnic groups had a variety of arrangements for interpreters: some relied on Social Services, other local hospital staff, family members or commercial interpreting services. Information on services and/or the Mental Health Act was available in a range of languages in all but one of the districts with large ethnic minority groups. However, this information was of variable quality. Some of the districts with smaller ethnic populations had also prepared leaflets, particularly on the Mental Health Act, in a variety of languages. Many Districts appeared to have commissioned their own translations of the documents produced centrally in English.

4.34   Two districts had appointed ethnic minority workers. One district was funding a black advocacy worker while the other had four link nurses working with the ethnic communities. These nurses were reported to be overwhelmed by demand for their services and were said not to be able to give enough time to people with severe or long term illness.

> **One trust employed two members of staff to provide advocacy for minority ethnic groups.**

Mental Health Act

Provider items in protocol: 3,11,17,25,27,66,95

4.35   Since Scotland has its own legislation and Northern Ireland operates under a Mental Health Order, ratings in Scottish and Northern Irish districts were made on the basis of practice equivalent to that in England. All districts indicated that they complied with the Act's requirements on the provision of standard information and letters (Section 133 of the Act).

4.36   Most districts reported that they currently audited the use of Section 117, or had done so in the past. In some cases it was not clear that the approach to audit was systematic or critical, or more than a simple enumeration of cases. In one district, a recently revised policy and procedure for implementing the Care Programme Approach contained an impressive proposal for regular auditing.

4.37 Virtually all districts reported no serious problems with availability of Approved Social Workers (ASWs) or Section 12 approved doctors. One district reported that delays for ASWs were longer during office hours, presumably because social workers had other duties. Another district reported that some delays occurred as an inevitable consequence of being a large rural district with long travelling times between sites.

4.38 All districts reported that there was a designated place of safety: either the local police station, or on NHS premises. In most cases the designation of the local police station appeared to cause no problem, but in two districts it did. In one of these, designation was objected to by the police. In the other, the police station was described in a recent Mental Health Act Commission report as 'a dreadful environment'. Examples of NHS provision included the A&E department, a District General Hospital - based in an acute psychiatric admission ward, and a hospital-based assessment clinic. In one district there appeared some uncertainty about the specific location of a Section 136 place of safety; the section had not been used in the preceding 12 months.

4.39 The requirement for the allocation of key workers for Section 117 patients was not met in all districts. In one, the deficiency had been put right and the imminent introduction of a new policy and procedure (for CPA, Section 117 and supervision registers) would assure good practice. In other districts, problems were compounded by those of CPA implementation, including statements that there were insufficient trained staff available to take on the key worker role. Several districts acknowledged that they did not strictly observe all the requirements of the Mental Health Act Code of Practice. In two districts there appeared to be very good examples of particular effort being taken to publicise and monitor the code.

4.40 Two districts appeared to have little or no difficulty in obtaining access to medium secure provision, probably because the need rarely arose. However most providers were concerned about poor patient care, potential or actual risk to other patients and staff, and diversion of resources to provide crisis care etc., caused by delays in obtaining places. These concerns were echoed by commissioners, since expensive ECRs were necessary when secure services were locally inadequate or non-existent.

In one district a Patient Administration System (PAS) included information on Section 117 patients with a triggering mechanism for scheduled reviews.

Violence

Provider items in protocol: 89,90,91,92,93

4.41 Violent incidents in the acute units of inner city districts were frequent, causing problems for other in-patients, as well as staff. The heavy demand on in-patient facilities was partly associated with social problems in inner city areas.

4.42 All but one district had policies for the management of violence and/or aggression. Violence was seen as a key issue in the acute wards and in most wards policies had been developed for these areas.

There were few policies specifically designed for staff in community settings. Nine of the eleven districts had policies and procedures in place to ensure that violent incidents were recorded separately from medical notes and that staff were debriefed following incidents.

4.43 The staff working in acute in-patient wards in all districts had received some training in the management of violence. This was mainly in 'breakaway', and control and restraint techniques. Two districts were also training their staff in risk assessment and 'de-escalation' techniques. In four districts staff in the community were receiving training in the management of violence. One of these districts had developed a standardised assessment of risk for patients referred to community services. Only one district ran training courses for medical staff.

In one district a specific budget was identified for 40 training places per annum; all staff could apply for these places.

Staff training

Provider item in protocol: 20

4.44 Many services either gave a low priority to post qualification training and development of all professionals, or tried to carry it out with inadequate budgets. Some practitioners appeared poorly trained or perhaps were poorly managed. A visitor with a nursing background commented that one CPN was trying to use transactional analysis as a helpful method of treatment for schizophrenia. There often appeared to be no strategy in planning training for individual professions, and no attempt at multidisciplinary training aimed at the clinical team. Nor were attempts made to prioritise training to match the declared priorities of the service. Multidisciplinary audit was insufficiently used to identify training needs. Innovative training programmes, such as the Thorn initiative, had yet to make any noticeable impact. The future dissemination of skills-based training programmes for all mental health professionals is therefore of great importance.

4.45 Limited clinical psychology input for the treatment of the severely mentally ill (both in direct work with patients and indirectly as consultants or trainers) was noticeable in most of the visits and was not simply a function of the numbers of psychologists employed by Trusts.

Chapter 5

Users & Carers

Introduction

5.1   Users' and carers' organisations were represented at the CSAG Conference in March 1994, where both the design of the project and a draft of the protocol were discussed. Many organisations subsequently sent useful written comments, both general and with specific reference to local district standards. During August, after the team visits, local branches were contacted in order to arrange meetings to discuss the local district services. Six such visits were made. Information was obtained by telephone or letter from the other five. The comments below reflect mainly local concerns. Users and carers were sometimes seen together, sometimes separately.

5.2   There was substantial agreement on most points between users and carers, and both tended to be more critical of standards than were providers. It should be recognised that the number of informants was low, and the comments reported are their own, not the judgements of an enquiry team.

Users

Influence on local services

5.3   In most districts there are committees through which users' views are intended to be represented. For example, a strategy group in one district is meant to provide a forum for the views of both users and carers; the latter, however, expressed the view, shared by other groups, that their comments were not acted upon. In another district it was suggested that only the official complaints procedure was effective in getting comments listened to - 'consultation' was a one-way process and did not mean involvement in action. In other districts, users felt that such committees were almost 'token gestures' on the part of the Trust and Health Authority, and reported having felt intimidated when they attended meetings. In another district there had been no mechanism at all but a first meeting was planned.

Access to information

5.4   Hospital managers have a duty under Section 132 of the Mental Health Act to provide written and oral information about patients' and nearest relatives' rights under the Act. Although a wide range of high quality information leaflets about illnesses and medication is produced, both locally and nationally, these are rarely available in out-patient departments or on wards. Some users reported having had to research topics such as medication alone or send off to national charities to obtain copies of leaflets. Some local charity offices were well stocked with information booklets, but were inaccessible to patients on a day-to-day basis. Information about the Mental Health Act and Tribunals was available only on the walls of acute wards in one district, or orally on wards in another. The latter had an excellent service directory but it was not available to users.

5.5   There were translated information booklets in the majority of the districts visited. In one district with a relatively high ethnic minority, one user complained that he could not get any translated information about his illness to give to his family. A translated document describing 'Your Rights Under The Mental Health Act 1983' was commonly available elsewhere, often translated locally and provided by individual districts at substantial expense (see paragraph 4.34).

5.6   It was generally felt that access to medical records was possible but not welcomed. One user claimed however that when he tried to obtain his records he was told that they had been lost. One patient who was refused access to a psychologist's report was granted it only after intervention by a local voluntary organisation.

Keyworker and CPA

5.7   None of the user informants in the districts visited was well informed about the Care Programme Approach. In one district, users knew the names of their keyworkers but were unclear about their functions and said they were very difficult to get hold of when needed. They sometimes had to wait weeks for an appointment. In another, neither of the two informants had a keyworker or knew what the term implied. However, in another district, there was an emergency telephone line to Social Services and keyworkers were described very positively by service users.

Emergency and crisis intervention

5.8   Emergency and crisis intervention in most districts was reported as 'ad hoc'. In one district it was difficult to get help from primary care and although one A&E department was helpful another was not. In another district an emergency line run by Social Services proved to be a helpful first point of contact; few had been told of the nationally available helplines or advisory services.

Care in an emergency

5.9   This item provoked most comment. Most acute wards were reported to consist of large noisy communal rooms, with little privacy or opportunity to avoid passive smoking. Single rooms were uncommon. Toilet and bathing facilities were usually adequate, although in one district men and women had to share a bathroom in one of the hospitals and toilet facilities were poor. In another district the acute wards were described as being dirty; at least one user had suffered an assault. In another district patients were commonly sent some distance away for care, a situation they found distressing. In another district the acute wards were described as dangerous, with harassment of female patients, regular incidents of theft, assault and sexual harassment. Short stay accommodation in another district was described by local carers as 'depressing, cramped and squalid'.

Residential accommodation and rehabilitation

5.10   The range of other residential accommodation was described as fair in three districts, although many reported long waiting lists. There was a complaint that staff in a hostel in another district were not interested in residents and did not take their needs seriously. Others described staff support as being very good.

5.11   Users reported a range of rehabilitation and other activities in several districts. Some called for additional advocacy and befriending schemes, more day centres, mental health resource centres, employment and pre-employment schemes and crisis centres. Users also complained about a lack of activities in the evenings or at the weekend. Some felt that the sheltered workshops offered were only suitable for very psychiatrically disabled people. In all districts, users identified a need for better advice about benefits, and many were reluctant to go back into full-time employment or voluntary work because they would lose benefits should things not work out.

Treatment and consultation

5.12   Users in most districts complained that 5-10 minute appointments with the consultant or the GP did not allow them enough time to discuss medical or personal problems in full or to ask all the questions that they might wish to. There was a general complaint about the lack of, or long wait for (12-18 months in one district), psychosocial intervention. Some users complained that their physical health problems were not taken seriously. In another district there was concern about the high turnover of psychiatrists with a resulting lack of continuity for the patient. Some, however, had experienced positive and successful sessions of family therapy.

Carers

Influence on local services

5.13   Few carers thought there was an effective channel for expressing their views about local health services. Carers in one district reported that, although they had been sent draft documents from their local trust, none of their comments had been acted on and they were not given an explanation for this. In another district carers felt that the trust had been selective in that they had consulted carers about community care plans but not about discharge policies or hospital closure. Many of the carers who took part in the study proved themselves to be important campaigners on the behalf of the mentally ill. Many felt that they deserved greater recognition by service providers and be given more opportunity to comment on the care of their relative and local service planning.

Access to information

5.14   Many carers reported having carried out their own research to find out about their relatives' illness and the side effects of medication. The lack of information reported by users was confirmed. Where service directories were available to staff they were not made available to carers.

Keyworker and CPA

5.15   In one district in particular, carers felt that it was too easy for those suffering from schizophrenia to slip through the care net. It was reported that having a keyworker was useful until the sufferer moved into another area. Better contact between carers and keyworkers could help to prevent this happening in some cases. Some patients had more than one keyworker. It was common in another district to have to wait several days to see a keyworker.

Care in an emergency

5.16   Carers reported a number of different methods for obtaining help in an emergency. Some praised the actions of the police and ambulance services. While others were able to obtain effective help from their GP, many relied on informal arrangements of their own. Most felt that much more could be done to improve emergency help. However, in one district, carers were alarmed at the proposed introduction of a mobile crisis intervention team because it was felt that, although it was essential for those in crisis to receive help quickly, the sudden presence of a number of unfamiliar people could cause the sufferer to take flight.

Respite care

5.17   In almost every district, carers reported a lack of effective and available respite care.

Treatment and consultation

5.18   In some districts carers felt that consultants often did not respect or listen to their views and also that they had little access to key personnel involved in their relatives' care, especially during stays in hospital. In one district local advocates reported an incident in which visitors to an acute ward had come to the conclusion that their relative was dead because they did not know that he had been put in seclusion. Many carers reported that they had been given either very short notice or no notice at all of their relatives' discharge from hospital. Family therapy was felt by many carers to be useful, although this and other psychosocial interventions were difficult to obtain.

5.19   Elderly relatives of people with schizophrenia were often worried about what would happen to the user when the carer died. Another concern was the degree to which users can be allowed to drop out of care, with no help from either health or social services.

5.20   Informal carers in the majority of the districts felt frustrated that their efforts were not obtaining the best possible care for their loved ones. For many carers the main burden of caring for a relative with schizophrenia was reported to be a financial one.

Chapter 6

Social Services

Introduction

6.1   In this chapter information from discussions with the social services departments in each of the districts visited (10 out of the 11) is presented. The meeting with social services sought their views on the current state of the organisation and quality of the health purchasers and providers visited by the CSAG team. A number of key issues were discussed with them which broadly can be classified under two headings: a) joint planning activity - the extent to which health and social services as commissioners have joint mechanisms to consult, plan and develop strategy; and b) operational working with health providers and how issues of working together (on, for example, the CPA, Section 117 of the MHA and care management) are being tackled. Problems specific to their locality were also discussed.

Joint planning

6.2   In all districts there is Social Services involvement in the preparation and implementation of joint purchasing and commissioning strategies. In most cases, however, these are at fairly early stages of development and have not yet had any significant impact on improving the quality and range of services available to people with schizophrenia or a severe mental illness. Joint planning, consultation and strategy are developing but only in a minority of cases so far do they influence community care planning. In one district there was a good example of a newly formed commissioning group linked into the community care planning process. In another district, however, health and social services were being developed separately.

6.3   Few Social Services authorities reported that joint commissioning and purchasing strategies had been agreed with health authorities and where particular developments had occurred they were mainly with providers in terms, for example, of the establishment of community mental health teams. Where joint planning arrangements had been developed successfully, agreements on purchasing strategies and responsibilities and levels of investment were having a positive impact on services. One district provided an example of a new joint mental health strategy developed by the Health Authority and Social Services, following consultation with local provider units, voluntary organisations, carers and service users. Even where joint planning is in the early stages of development there are examples of closer collaboration in terms of particular initiatives, e.g. in the development of services for mentally disordered offenders.

6.4   Some Social Services authorities reported difficulties in developing with health purchasers joint approaches to service delivery. In one district, there was concern that a hospital closure programme was being negotiated without consultation with Social Services. These difficulties tended to show up in the implementation of the CPA, Section 117, care management, and the impact on after care services, and were exacerbated where there were no strong commissioning arrangements, with health providers taking the lead in planning sod implementing change. In one district, however, there were examples of joint policies in place for the integration of the CPA, care management, hospital discharge, Section 117 and planning.

6.5   Social Services authorities had identified the issues that they believed needed action. Their lead role in community care planning gives them particular responsibilities for ensuring that the necessary community support services are in place and for working closely with health purchasers to agree the strategies and funding arrangements to secure them. More is known about needs and there is evidence of increased investment by Social Services under the new community care arrangements. This is not yet however in most cases integrated with health purchasing strategies.

Operational arrangements

6.6   Social Services authorities reported similar variations in operational arrangements with providers. There is evidence of closer working relationships with NHS Trust staff, particularly in the development of community mental health teams, but in many cases there is insufficient integration in the management, delivery and provision of services. In one district there was an example of good multi-disciplinary working within a Community Mental Health Team.

6.7   In a few districts, there are agreed operational arrangements within which Health and Social Services staff are working together closely. Joint policies and procedures for CPA and care management have been drawn up which assist hospital discharge and individual care plans.

6.8   There are some individual examples of collaborative work to co-ordinate and improve the arrangements for the care of people with a severe mental illness. In one case, care managers are piloting work with those with the most complex needs. They are funded by Social Services and managed by Health. In another example, community mental health nurses are being trained jointly with Social Services staff as assessors for care management.

6.9   In one district where there are strong links between Social Services and both the health purchasers and the providers, residential and day services have been set up and are managed in close collaboration. In this district there are also close links with housing authorities and the effect is believed to minimise the number of individuals who fall through the network of care.

6.10   Most Social Services authorities recognised the need to consider organisational changes in response to the changing nature of mental health services. In most districts, work was in hand to match staffing arrangements with the creation of mental health teams. In one or two cases this was proving difficult, especially where Social Services neighbourhood teams did not comprise staff in the community with specialist mental health skills. This has a significant impact on after-care as the specialist staff based in local acute units cannot continue to supervise discharged patients indefinitely. In general, however, Social Services authorities recognised their staff required specialist skills to work effectively in community mental health teams.

6.11   In some cases, Social Services authorities acknowledged insufficient attention to the care programme approach and supervision registers. This was primarily attributed to the absence of consultation or involvement in the development of policies and procedures for implementation.

6.12   A number of Social Services authorities expressed concern on these issues:

- the transition from hospital to community based care and the extent to which sufficient funds are or will be available to develop and sustain the services required now and in the future

- the extent to which services in the community (including local hospital units) are being targeted on those with schizophrenia and severe mental illness

- the availability of appropriate long-term supported accommodation in the community for those who do not require specialised residential/hospital care

- the arrangements for the care of those with high levels of needs who are difficult to manage, including mentally disordered offenders

- the extent to which the care programme approach is being applied effectively and the lack of joint work in integrating this with local authority responsibilities for Section 117 Mental Health Act 1983 and care management

- the need for direction by DoH as to who should select and authorise the key worker - Health or Social services, and who in either service

- the accessibility of specialist mental health workers to support Social Services staff in residential and day services and in the community as a whole.

Comment by visiting teams

6.13 Many of the standards considered by teams that visited NHS units should involve close links between the health and social services. Comments by members generally echoed those recorded above. In some districts there were few effective links. Problems were seen at their worst when neither service gave sufficient priority to people with severe mental illness to counter the possibility that the less severely ill may be more articulate in their demand for services. Despite difficulties, however, there were districts where the two professional groups were working together in an effective and impressive way.

Chapter 7

Conclusions

Introduction

7.1   The study was completed rapidly, was based on short visits to a small sample of Districts, and could offer only a snapshot taken at one point within what should be a cycle of audit, action and follow-up. One of our main recommendations is that Version 1 of the protocol should be revised, the methodology refined and the study repeated. Our initial study might be regarded as a substantial pilot for wider use of a revised protocol.

7.2   Nevertheless, we suggest that tentative conclusions can be based on the results, which were in line with those of recent surveys using other methods. Our conclusions are informed by, but do not rely exclusively on, analysis of ratings for twenty key points. These scorings, and the rankings by aggregate scores, were used primarily to help us think about the characteristics of good, average and low-scoring districts. In paragraphs 7.3-7.15 we consider these comparative characteristics; and in paragraphs 7.16-7.28 we review our findings against our specific terms of reference.

Comparative Characteristics

Socio-economic factors

7.3   We were interested to note (see 4.7) that there appeared to be no relationship between the socio-economic factors and total scores. District A was more rural than most of the others and members of the visiting team were of the opinion that it would be difficult to reproduce such standards with the same resources in an urban district such as G. However, district H was rural and small but, some good clinical standards notwithstanding, did not come high in the rankings.

Morale and leadership

7.4   The term 'morale' sums up many of the differences that could be discerned between the three groups of districts. The main elements are: shared vision between purchaser and provider; commitment to clear aims and achievable targets; shared audit and accountability between professions and managers; organisational stability; and strong clinical leadership. Clinical leadership in particular might be promoted by giving greater priority to severe mental illness within psychiatric trainees' general and higher professional training, including theoretical and practical management of patients and the different systems of treatment and provision of care.

7.5   Low morale districts are characterised by a lack of these features. If there is no informed and sympathetic interaction between Chief Executives of purchasing and providing bodies, if clinical staff do not feel involved in making decisions about the development of their services and have no control over the demands of their job, if there is a state of constant flux with frequent management changes and a high staff turnover, and if the resources are inadequate to achieve acceptable standards of care, the organisation becomes demoralised and falls apart. A high quality service develops gradually over time; it cannot be created overnight by administrative fiat.

7.6   We believe these features can be identified, and should be expanded into a revised protocol. Accordingly we comment on them at more length in Appendix 3.

Central policy guidelines

7.7   Central policy guidelines, like clinical guidelines, need to be seen as relevant locally before they are welcomed as part of everyday clinical and administrative work. Two examples are the Care Programme Approach (CPA) and guidance on co-operation between health and social care agencies.

7.8   None of the eight English districts visited had fully implemented CPA three years after its introduction. Most users and carers we spoke to did not know what it was. In some cases the Department had been told that implementation was complete. If this sample is characteristic, the challenge for the service and the Health Departments is to ensure that all relevant and necessary policies are implemented. Supervision Registers and the Power of Supervised Discharge will raise similar problems, since they would be subsets of the CPA.

7.9   Separate CPA and care management policies, and often separately managed teams working with the same user or carer, compound problems at the interface between the NHS and Social Services. Collaboration or lack of it depends on personal relationships at several different levels. Among the most senior staff, relationships work better but a clearer structure is needed to spread trust and collaboration throughout both organisations. Organisational arrangements that serve to facilitate joint working were seen in Northern Ireland and Wales. In Northern Ireland, health and social services are part of a single Board; staff roles were clear and there was no professional isolation or friction. In Wales, the All Wales Strategy for Mental Health gives direction and advice to local planning, including close collaboration between health authorities, primary care and social services. The Department of Health has issued for consultation new draft guidance on inter-agency co-operation but this was not available at the time of our visits.

Models of care

7.10   All districts visited were still in various stages of transition away from a model of care for the severely mentally ill based on a sheltered relatively closed community and towards one in which provisions are diverse, local and dispersed, domestic in size and appearance, and relying on teamwork and good communications to maintain continuity of care. The objective remains to provide all the functions of 'asylum': physical care; housing; occupation; recreation; graduated protection; companionship; 24 hour help in crises, without the need to assemble all these functions on a single site. The aim is to increase choice and autonomy. The evidence from experimental projects, such as TAPS (Team for the Assessment of Psychiatric Services) is that focused provisions for most of the long-term residents resettled from the large hospitals have been acceptable, though there remains a sizable group with special needs. Assuming that such provisions can be made for all the present long-term residents, the problem that chiefly exercises planners of mental health services is that of people who have become ill more recently.

7.11   The services visited, particularly in their community aspects, were in transition between models of care (also see Audit Commission Report); some were in turmoil. The two chief models are centred on primary care or on Community Mental Health Teams (CMHTs). In the former, some specialist staff are incorporated into the primary team; in the latter they are separate but theoretically in close communication.

7.12 The primary care model is close to the prevalence in the general population but, by the same token, may miss the wood for the trees since less severe disorders appear more frequently than severe mental illness, with a possible drift of staff attention away from the latter. If so, there would be less peer support for the specialists and, a danger of becoming cut off from the rest of the mental health service. There is also a danger that specialists succeed in integrating with some primary care teams better than with others.

7.13 CMHTs have to work across organisational barriers, including those between health and social care mentioned in 7.9. Elsewhere, examples were seen in a few districts of social workers functioning as full members of community health teams, but this was not the norm. Close liaison between Community Mental Health Teams and all local GPs is important.

Variations in service

7.14 Wide variations between districts mean that people with a severe mental illness are given a different quality of service depending on where they live, and even within a given locality where there is sectorisation.

Communications and audit

7.15 Some, perhaps many, of the factors described above would be easier to put into practice for subsequent audit if a better infrastructure of communications were in place. The following procedures would facilitate the process of audit and follow up:

(a) A shorter and more manageable protocol based on an assessment of the key points;

(b) Detailed audit standards based on professional guidance and incorporated in the new protocol;

(c) Use of outcomes scales in contracts;

(d) The 'national' statistics available to districts are limited to service volumes and are of little use for measuring outcomes. It was difficult to collect even these minimal statistics from districts and interpreting what was available was questionable. High quality data are essential for purchasing and providing health care.

(e) Population based needs assessment was perhaps rated too generously in most districts and more specific guidelines are required.

(f) Simple and user-friendly CPA registers, including Supervision and Supervised Discharge Registers as subsets, should be funded, set up and piloted in a broad range of districts. Both paper-based and computerised systems are acceptable so long as they work in practice. They should be developed not only for their specific impact on continuity of good clinical care but because they are mental health information systems in embryo.

40

Fulfilling the Remit

7.16   The remit given to CSAG (see 1.2 above) was in general to advise on standards of clinical care for people with a diagnosis of schizophrenia, and in particular to review existing clinical standards, how these were reflected in contracts and whether they were met by providers, and measures in place to achieve a seamless service.

Review of existing standards

7.17   Our multidisciplinary panel of experts found no comprehensive statement of standards, but collated for CSAG those guidelines and standards it believed would command professional support. Our study protocol was based on these, and amended following a CSAG conference and two pilot visits (see Chapter 3). Use in eleven districts showed it to be generally robust and sensitive enough for its purpose. The Protocol has now been revised and shortened in the light of this experience, and is available as Volume 2 of this report.

Are standards reflected in contracts?

7.18   No purchaser had specified clinical standards for schizophrenia in contracts with providers. Several mentioned severe mental illness but only one had developed a full strategic plan, based on local needs assessment and involvement of clinicians and others concerned, which identified and targeted the needs of severely mentally ill people. This district's contracts did not mention schizophrenia specifically and it is questionable whether it is necessary to do so separately from severe mental illness.

Are standards met by providers?

7.19   All the items in the protocol for providers are in some way linked to the treatment and care of people with schizophrenia or other severe mental illnesses and are described in chapters 4.27-51. The top-scoring district achieved a mean of 2.75 for the first eleven provider key points, not quite reaching 3 ('good'). The equivalent mean for the lowest scoring district was 0.90; better than 0, which would mean 'not met at all', but not quite reaching 1 ('poor').

7.20   The essence of the audit approach is to try to improve the average level of performance and to continue as that average improves. It would be unrealistic to expect uniformly high standards in districts at present. Overall, however, the general level of performance is disappointing and should be substantially improved. This conclusion is relieved by striking examples of good practice scattered across all districts including the two lowest-scoring ones. The audit principle requires that these strong points be recognised and copied by other districts whilst, at the same time, priorities are set in order to raise the level of care where it fails to meet other standards.

Were standards audited in order to achieve a seamless service?

7.21   The third part of the remit specifies three topics for special attention: audit against clinical standards, including diagnosis and assessment; the Care Programme Approach; and inter-agency working to produce a seamless service.

Clinical standards, diagnosis and assessment

7.22 Full clinical guidelines for each aspect of clinical care, for example detailed medication or rehabilitation regimes, were not included in the protocol since quality assurance of these aspects is a matter for individual clinical audit and is impossible to assess during a brief team visit.

7.23 The topic of diagnosis was indeed found to be important. All members of the multidisciplinary visiting teams and the Schizophrenia Committee agreed that the term 'schizophrenia', when used to designate the presence of specific and definable experiences and behaviours associated with distress, impairment, or risk of harm to self or others, is an essential element in the process of assessment, in order to prescribe an appropriate plan of care for an individual (see Chapter 2).

7.24 Members of the teams who had nursing qualifications were particularly concerned that CPNs in some districts were unwilling to use the term 'schizophrenia' because they regarded it as stigmatising. Item 76 of the Version 1 Protocol specifically addressed the issue of priority for severe mental illness. Five of eleven districts did not prioritise and CPNs had a relatively low proportion of such vulnerable patients on their caseloads. This also tended to be true when the chief attachment was to general practice. This, therefore, could be a serious hindrance to the provision of a seamless service for the severely mentally ill.

Care Programme Approach (CPA)

7.25 Assessment more broadly is considered as part of the CPA, which is specifically addressed in 7.7–8 above. The ideas behind the CPA are good and well expressed in written Department of Health guidelines. The districts in N.Ireland and Wales could not be assessed since the CPA applies only to England and Scotland. Every English district had some kind of paper record system but in seven out of eight these did not appear to work: practitioners often did not understand the principles and many had reservations about top-down imposition, bureaucracy, cumbersome application, confidentiality and lack of resources for implementation. Users and carers had even less understanding of the system. All this adds up to lack of ownership, and suggests that the success or failure of Supervision Registers and Supervised Discharge will depend on similar factors.

Interagency working

7.26 Joint commissioning of mental health services, whether between district and GP fundholders or district and social services, was conspicuous by its absence. The care provided for the severely mentally ill by the primary and secondary health services and the social services, particularly in the eight English districts, is far from seamless. However it was not possible within the timescale to visit GP practices or to interview any GP fundholders and our comments about, for example, the priority GPs allocated to severely ill people are mainly from the perspective of those in the Secondary Sector.

7.27 Collaboration with Social Services was tenuous in most districts. An equivalent problem to 'labelling' meant that the philosophy of care often differed from that in the health services. The Northern Ireland example demonstrates that the barriers are not insurmountable. Users and carers complained that they were allowed no influence on planning and management, and felt frustrated by the token nature of the few contacts they did have. Seamlessness should be for their benefit but if it is lacking they feel the lack most.

42

7.28 The adoption of a common data set by all those involved in serving severely mentally ill people would facilitate multi-disciplinary and multi-professional audit, and would help to improve both the practice and monitoring of overlapping services.

Scope for further enquiries

7.29 The study was in effect a pilot of the Version 1 protocol, In it's revised form, Version 2, the protocol needs to be more widely used further to improve it and broaden its ownership by local clinicians, managers and commissioners. Particular attention should be paid to the contribution that users and carers can make. Further development of the protocol should also take account of the experience of other countries in the European Community, Australia, Canada and the USA where work similar to CSAG's is mooted or already being undertaken.

7.30 The revised, Version 2, protocol and method could be used in further local audits that not only provide an assessment of services but lead to local policies for improvement. Follow-up would then continue the audit cycle by assessing outcomes and once again considering priorities in the light of the results. This would in time become a routine part of district procedures.

7.31 Monitoring the performance of purchasers is the responsibility of NHS Executives. In England this is undertaken by Regional Offices. These and other monitoring bodies such as the Health Advisory Service, Social Services Inspectorate and Audit Commission may find the protocol a useful adjunct to other methods of assessing performance, with the NHS Executive Headquarters overseeing progress in England and applying lessons from these assessments.

Chapter 8 | Recommendations

CSAG was asked to advise on standards for people with schizophrenia and in particular to review existing clinical standards, how these were reflected in contracts, whether they were met by providers, the effectiveness of audit including diagnosis and assessment, the Care Programme Approach and the interface with social care. The preceding chapters set out the findings of and conclusions from our reviews; the following summarises our recommendations to improve standards in the light of those findings.

1   The Version 2 protocol should be further developed through wider use by clinicians, managers and commissioners as part of their local audit measures

2   Commissioners should after consulting users and carers, agree with service providers explicit statements of the standards to be achieved locally, and consider referring in these statements to use of the Version 2 protocol, as developed, as one of the methods of auditing clinical and managerial aspects of the district service.

3   The NHS Executive should, where it has serious concerns about standards and the effectiveness of local audit to identify weaknesses, consider using the Version 2 protocol itself or inviting an independent agency to investigate in more detail.

4   The place of skilled diagnosis within the clinical and social assessment of people with severe mental illness in indicating priority for services should be recognised in contracts, supported and audited.

5   A simple register system should be developed to support the information requirements of the Care Programme Approach, with Supervision Registers and Supervised Discharge as subsets, and to underpin clinical work with high priority groups and clinical audit.

6   The principles of multi-disciplinary and multi-professional audit should be applied in all agencies providing care for designated groups such as the severely mentally ill. This will require harmonisation of methods of data collection by local mental health teams, general practices and social services.

7   CSAG should repeat its district surveys, following discussion with districts regarding the visiting teams' assessments of standards and priorities for change.

Version 1 Protocol Used by the Visiting Teams – April 1994

Introduction

It is assumed that the District Health Authority sets the standards for, and maintains up-to-date information about, a geographically defined population.

The standards have been drafted in the spirit of audit, as a basis for discussion and modification,

without any assumption that perfect standards can be reached throughout the health and social services.

However, average care can be improved by regular monitoring, and virtually all health services professionals, whether clinical or administrative, do wish to improve care.

The standards set out in the CSAG-S Protocol are either:

- in the form of positive statements that are relatively simple to affirm or deny, with supporting evidence if requested;
- or quantified more precisely, on the assumption that such information is normally available to purchasers and providers.

Most items can be rated on one or both of two scales:

- the extent to which the standard has been achieved;
- the rapidity with which the service can be made available.

Both scales can be checked on a list in order to measure progress year by year.

Evidence is required to show that positive answers are justified. There will undoubtedly be negative answers that will provide a challenge to purchasers and providers when considering priorities for the future.

Although the protocol deals specifically with schizophrenia, the principles apply to services for all people aged 18 or more with a severe mental illness. Children's services and specialised services for substance disorders, dementia and learning disabilities are excluded.

Part 1: PURCHASER – Purchaser Provider Interaction

This information, amplified by the Team's local discussions, shows that the Purchaser's strategy identifies:

1   Problems specifically characteristic of SCZ
2   Problems of SMI
3   Separate targets for SCZ and/or SMI
4   The characteristics of and interactions between statutory health providers and LASS providers
5   The characteristics of and interactions between statutory health providers and voluntary and non-statutory providers
6   Local socio-demographic factors that should influence service planning for SMI

The Purchaser's service specification:

7   Is based on a thorough appraisal of national and local information relevant to needs assessment
8   Is based on full consultation with relevant parties
9   Is realistic in the local context
10   Includes a comprehensive range of services for people with SMI

The Provider's business plan(s):

11   This Provider does have a business plan
12   Specifies realistic intentions for services and facilities for people with SMI/SCZ
13   Has been used in negotiation with the Purchaser when drawing up the contract

Contract(s) between this Purchaser and this Provider:

14   Block, cost & volume, activity limited block, other specify
15   There is an explicit contract for services for SCZ
16   There is an explicit contract for services for SMI/SCZ

The contract specifies the following currencies:

17   FCEs
18   Patient Bed Days
19   Out-patient activity
20   Other activity indicators – specify
21   Care protocols – specify
22   Outcome indicators – specify
23   Other – specify

Implementation and Quality:

The contract specifies and requires implementation of:

24   The Care Programme Approach
25   Care Management

26   Section 117, MHA

27   A Supervision Registrar from April 1994.

28   A Quality Assurance strategy for SCZ/SMI

29   Health of the Nation targets

30   The Patients Charter targets

31   Quality Assurance protocols

32   Quality is the responsibility of a named Director

33   Annual targets are published and circulated widely

Clinical audit:

The Provider has explicit mechanisms in place for:

34   Regular clinical audit

35   Regular medical audit

36   Written records of audit sessions

37   Audit protocols to guide procedures

38   Specific protocols for SCZ

39   Specific protocols for SMI

40   Ensuring that audit decisions change practices

41   Ensuring that audit decisions change services

Perverse incentives:

42   Perverse incentives are not apparent in the commissioning process or contract set

General statements:

43   Is the contract developed in the spirit of joint commissioning?

44   How is the Purchaser/Provider split working?

Part II: PROVIDER – Description of District Services

1. Continuity of Care and Communication

1.1 Involvement of patient/client and informal carer

Patients/clients and informal carers are involved in service planning both individually and group, and have mechanisms for commenting on outcomes of care and how services meet their needs:

1	National Schizophrenia Fellowship or other carer groups	Scale I: 0-4
2	Local Mental Health Associations (MIND)/other user groups	Scale I: 0-4
3	Patients/clients and informal carers have information specific to their different needs to facilitate access to support and services	Scale I: 0-4

1.2 Primary care liaison:

Mental health service staff work with local GPs to develop a liaison strategy, including:

4	Service directories are provided for primary care teams	Y/N
5	Practices which provide care for local residential facilities are encouraged by CMHT(s) to develop expertise in mental health problems.	Scale I: 0-4
6	CMHT(s) have regular meetings with general practices	Scale I: 0-4
7	Joint primary-secondary audit activities are carried out	Scale I: 0-4

1.3 Mental health record systems:

8   The district has a specialist mental health record system that effectively supports basic service functions. Best described as:

A fully integrated specialist computerised mental health record system
A partially integrated computerised mental health record system
Some computerised stand alone system(s) to support specific functions
A paper based system alone

A system records individuals subject to:

9	the Care Programme Approach	Computerised/Paper/None
10	the Supervision Register	Computerised/Paper/None
11	Section 117 of the Mental Health Act	Computerised/Paper/None
12	All computerised systems provide adequate checks to prevent unauthorised access, and fully preserve confidentiality	Y/N

A system provides up to date information about the needs and care of those with SMI at risk of relapse, as follows:

13	includes the identity of all primary and specialist workers involved in care, and specifically the key worker	Y/N
14	includes referral letters, problem profile, care plan, review dates, outcome, discharge summary.	All/most/some/none
15	enables authorised information to be shared when responsibility is transferred from one health care worker to another	Scale I: 0-4
16	provides a basis for creating a district wide mental health information system, to underpin clinical care, audit, management, planning and statistics.	Scale I: 0-4

1.4 Local health service audit procedures:

Audit topics include:

17	Discharge planning to meet the requirements of the Care Programme Approach and Section 117	Y/N
18	Service co-ordination to ensure that care plans derived from assessment of need are carried through	Y/N

19   Systematic audits to monitor the quality of routine clinical care, learning
      from the study of 'adverse events', monitoring statistics relevant to
      promulgated audit guidelines   All\Most\Some\None

1.5 Education of mental health practitioners:

20   Education and training is provided and updated through routine audit,
      refresher courses, and exchanges between different agencies and/or settings   Y/N

1.6 A Service Directory:

21   Lists all local service settings and facilities for people with
      SCZ/SMI. Available to all workers, and to users and carers.   Y/N

2. Crisis and Emergency Intervention

22   There is appropriate hospital accommodation for the
      assessment of people referred for assessment in a psychiatric crisis   Scale I: 0-4
23   Such assessments are carried out by qualified and experienced workers   Scale I: 0-4
24   An outreach service can respond rapidly in
      emergency to provide help in domiciliary or other settings   Scale II: 0-7
25   Approved social workers are readily available for Mental Health Act assessments   Scale II: 0-7
26   Second medical opinions are readily available for Mental Health Act assessments   Scale II: 0-7
27   There is a place of safety for those subject to S136   Y\N

3. Residential Services and Facilities

A full range of services and facilities as specified below is available to every person with schizophrenia and to carers.

3.1 Short-stay hospital care (in general, less than 3 months):

28   Separate accommodation for 'intensive care' is available for those whose
      behaviour is temporarily threatening, self-harming or severely overactive   Scale II: 0-7
29   Staff ratios are such that 'challenging behaviour' can be controlled
      humanely and without undue disturbance to others residents on the ward   Y/N
30   Residents have opportunities for occupational therapy and recreation   True/False
31   No patient is resident on the acute ward simply because appropriate
      alternatives are lacking   True/False
32   No patient who needs aftercare is discharged without
      a plan of care and assured means of implementing it   True/False
33   Overall rating on quality of short-stay hospital care   Poor\Average\Good:0-4

3.2 Longer-term wards or hostel wards (in general, over 3 months):

34   Places are available for people whose behaviour or poor living skills mean that
      they need constant supervision; in particular from trained staff on duty at night   Scale II: 0-7

35	The accommodation is domestic in style	Y/N
36	A variety of daytime activities is available	Y/N
37	Residents have access to private outdoor space	Y/N
38	Overall rating on quality of longer-term ward care	Poor\Average\Good:0-4

3.3 Secure longer-term accommodation:

Accommodation is available for people who pose a danger to others and/or require intensive care for a longer period than would be appropriate for an intensive care ward.

39	Local security: e.g. a high-staffed unit	Scale II: 0-7
40	The accommodation is domestic in style	Y/N
41	A variety of daytime activities is available	Y/N
42	Medium security: e.g. Regional Secure Unit	Scale II: 0-7
43	High security: e.g. Special Hospital	Scale II: 0-7
44	Overall rating on quality of local secure accommodation care	Poor\Average\Good:0-4

3.4 Other residential accommodation:

A range of residential accommodation is available to cover the needs of people who do not require hostel-ward care.

45	Short stay accommodation with sleep-in and day staff	Scale II: 0-7
	Overall rating on quality of accommodation	Poor\Average\Good:0-4
46	Long-stay accommodation with sleep-in and day staff	Scale II: 0-7
	Overall rating on quality of accommodation	Poor\Average\Good:0-4
47	Day staffed accommodation	Scale II: 0-7
	Overall rating on quality of accommodation	Poor\Average\Good:0-4
48	Group homes or similar with up to daily visiting	Scale II: 0-7
	Overall rating on quality of accommodation	Poor\Average\Good:0-4
49	Group homes or similar with on-call facilities only	Scale II: 0-7
	Overall rating on quality of accommodation	Poor\Average\Good:0-4
50	Bed-sits or lodgings with supervised standards	Scale II: 0-7
	Overall rating on quality of accommodation	Poor\Average\Good:0-4
51	Respite facilities to allow users or carers a planned period away from stressful or tiring situations	Scale II: 0-7
	Overall rating on quality of accommodation	Poor\Average\Good:0-4
52	Care directed specifically at homeless and roofless people	Y/N
53	Care directed specifically at young persons (<18 years old)	Y/N

4. Day Services: Rehabilitation and Activity

People with SCZ/SMI, including those in residential and day settings, have access to the following opportunities:

54	Plenty of activities (available evenings and weekends), both structured (e.g. activity groups, sports at local centres) and unstructured (e.g. lunch and social clubs, outings, drop-in centre)	Scale I: 0-4
55	Education and training centres, e.g. basic numeracy and literacy classes, easy access to Adult Education facilities	Scale I: 0-4
56	Personal and domestic skills training, development and experience:	Scale I: 0-4
57	Work experience through rehabilitation, sheltered workshops, work-based projects, voluntary work and links with local industry:	Scale I: 0-4
58	Advocacy/befriending schemes	Y/N
59	Information about telephone helplines	Y/N

The following local day settings are available:

60	Day hospital	Scale II: 0-7
61	Day centre	Scale II: 0-7
62	Rehabilitation/pre-employment training workshops	Scale II: 0-7
63	Sheltered workshop	Scale II: 0-7
64	Places in local industry	Scale II: 0-7
65	Lunch or social club, drop-in centre	Scale II: 0-7

5. Care Programme Approach and Outreach

66   All those on the local active list, including those subject to the requirements of the Care Programme Approach (CPA) and Section 117 are allocated a key worker   Y/N

Care Programme Approach:

67	There is a written policy	Y/N
68	Specify grade of administrator	
69	% on CPA register with named keyworker	___%
70	% on CPA register with stated review date	___%

The intensive support and outreach service (case management):

71	Provides or co-ordinates comprehensive needs assessment meeting the requirements of CPA	Y/N
72	Develops, with the patient/client and carer, individual care plans that address the full range of needs	Y/N
73	Co-ordinates the delivery of care as agreed in the care plan and holds regular reviews	Y/N
74	Offers support to relatives and other 'informal' carers including respite care.	Y/N
75	Limits the case load of those working with the most disabled group to allow reasonable time for their needs	Y/N
76	People with schizophrenia and severe mental illness are given priority on active team lists	Y/N

6. Mental Health Interventions

77   The health and care needs of people with SCZ/SMI are subject to regular multidisciplinary review Y/N

The full range of interventions shown to have been effective in the care of people with SCZ/SMI are realistically available in practice:

78   Regular assessment and care for physical ill-health   Y/N
79   Regular monitoring and review of medication by skilled practitioners   Y/N
80   Access to medication shown to be beneficial for people
      who are otherwise treatment resistant (e.g. Clozapine)   Y/N
81   A full range of cognitive and behavioural therapies is offered for the relief and
      self-management of distressing symptoms, impaired functioning and adverse self-attitudes   Y/N
82   Specific family interventions aimed at relapse prevention   Y/N
83   Information and education is provided aimed at
      recognising and preventing the risk of relapse in those living alone   Y/N

7. Special Issues

7.1 Ethnic and cultural issues:

84   There is a good relationship with local community leaders   Y/N
85   Special care is taken to keep families fully informed   Y/N
86   Diagnoses are made with full appreciation of cultural
      factors that may complicate a diagnosis of schizophrenia: Scale I: 0-4
87   Particular care is taken when the possibility of using a section of the MHA arises: Y/N
88   All relevant CMHTs have available and use relevant expertise,
      e.g. free access to an interpreting service and specialist advice on cultural issues   Y/N

7.2 Prevention of violence and self-harm:

89   The risk of violence (dangerousness) is always considered
      during the assessment of people with severe mental illness   Y/N
90   Violent incidents are recorded in confidential records other than patients' notes   Y/N
91   All incidents of suicide and serious self harm are subject to audit review   Y/N
92   Staff in mental health teams are trained in the management of
      violent situations   All/Most/Some/None
93   Units at particular risk of violence are designed with its prevention and management in mind   Y/N
94   All staff are trained in the management of suicidal patients and
      serious self harm   All/Most/Some/None

7.3 Medicolegal issues:

95   The code of practice of the Mental Health Act is strictly adhered to   Y/N
96   No mentally ill people are held in prison through lack of mental health service alternatives Y/N
97   A diversion service is available at the local magistrates' court   Y/N
98   A 'bail hostel' or equivalent is available for mentally ill people   Y/N

99   There are good communications between CMHTs, social services,
      probation officers, the police, and local, regional and national secure units   Y/N

Rating Scales Used in Protocol

Two scales are used frequently throughout the CSAG-S protocol. One provides an estimate of the progress that has been made towards achieving the standard. The other is an approximate indicator of how rapidly a request for a given service can be met.

In some cases, it may be considered that it is inappropriate even to try to meet the standard; for example because there is disagreement as to its value, or because local circumstances make it inappropriate. In such cases, rate 9 and specify the reason.

Scale 1

What steps have been taken towards meeting the quality standard?
0.   No action yet taken (why not?)
1.   Active discussions with relevant parties
2.   Standard is partially met
3.   Standard is substantially met
4.   Standard is fully met
9.   Not known or not applicable (specify)
Specify, i.e. provide sufficient information to justify the rating chosen

Scale 2

If an authorised care worker requested the specified service today, how long would a patient or client wait before it became available?
0.   No such service available
1.   1 year +
2.   3-12 months
3.   1-3 months
4.   1-4 weeks
5.   1-7 days
6.   <24 hours
7.   <1 hour
9.   Not known or not applicable (specify)
Specify, i.e. provide sufficient information to justify the rating chosen

Quality of Residential Accommodation

Overall rating of the quality of each kind of residential accommodation.

Take into account non-clinical aspects of care environment: e.g. private (bathing and toilet facilities), single rooms, small scale domestic, comfortable, fosters independence.

Quality of staff-patient interaction.

Quality of personal/social interaction e.g. personalised care, consultation with users, supports autonomy, institutional routines flexible, occupation and time off wards.

Ratings of Version 1 Protocol Items for Providers

A2.1 Several methods of rating individual items were used:

A	Yes/No (Y/N)	the standard is met or not
B	True/False (T/F)	the standard statement is agreed to be true or false
C	Scale 1 (0 – 4)	indicates the degree to which the standard has been met
D	Scale 2 (0 – 7)	indicates whether a particular service exists, and if so, how long it would normally take to be made available
E	Quality rating (0 – 4) subscale used to rate the quality of residential accommodation	
F	All/Most/Some/None	
G	Computer/Paper/None	
X	Suggested scoring system inadequate and currently under review.	

A2.2 For scales 1 and 2 the mean score for the eleven districts is included. For those items rated by letter, the most frequently occurring response (described as the mode) has been recorded. A '-' appearing in a cell indicates that data is missing for that district. In some districts where more than one unit was rated, the rating may not be a whole number.

A2.3 Table 7 shows the ratings for each provider in numerical order. The method of rating (A-G; see A2.1 above) is shown after the item number in the first column. For Scales 1 and 2 (C and D) the mean district rating is shown in the last column. Full details of the statistical analysis (including the two blocks of items rated on scale 2) will be presented in Volume 2 together with the revised protocol.

A2.4 Because three provider items were difficult to rate in districts in Northern Ireland, Scotland and Wales, average ratings have been inserted. Relevant calculations are not affected when repeated omitting these items.

Table 7 Ratings on provider items in protocol

Item	Scale	A	B	C	D	E	F	G	H	I	J	K	Mean
1	C	3	2	3	3	1	1	1	2	1	3	2	2
2	C	2.5	2	3	4	1	1	3	2	2	2	2	2.23
3	C	3	3	3	2	2	3	2	4	3	3	2	2.73
4	A	Y	N	N	N	T	T	N	T	N	N	N	
5	C	1.5	–	3	2	0	0	2	2	1	1	0	1.25
6	C	1.5	2	1	2	2	0	2	2	0	0	–	1.25
7	C	2	2	3	2	0	0	2	0	0	0	0	1
8	X	–	–	–	–	–	–	–	–	–	–	–	
9	G	P	P	P	P	P	–	P	N	P	N	P	
10	G	P	P	N	N	N	N	N	C	P	N	P	
11	G	P	P	N	P	N	N	P	P	P	P	P	
12	A	N	Y	Y	Y	Y	Y	Y	Y	N	Y	Y	
13	A	Y	Y	Y	N	N	Y	Y	Y	Y	N	Y	
14	F	A	M	S	N	N	M	S	A	A	S	S	
15	C	3	4	2	1	0	3	2	4	2	1	2	2.18
16	C	2	1	2	1	0	2	2	1	1	1	0	1.18
17	A	Y	Y	Y	Y	N	Y	Y	Y	Y	N	N	
18	A	Y	Y	Y	Y	N	N	Y	N	N	N	N	
19	F	M	S	M	M	S	M	M	S	S	S	A	
20	C	2	2	3	2	3	3	2	2	3	2	0	2.18
21	A	Y	N	N	Y	N	Y	N	Y	N	N	N	
22	C	3.5	3	4	2	2	4	3	2	4	2	2	2.86
23	C	4	4	4	3	3	4	3	4	4	3	2	3.45
24	D	6	0	6	6	6	6	5	6	6	7	0	4.91
25	D	6	6	6	6	6	6	6	6	6	7	6	6.1
26	D	6	6	–	6	6	5	6	5	6	6	6	5.8
27	A	Y	Y	Y	Y	Y	Y	Y	Y	Y	Y	Y	
28	D	7	7	6	–	0	7	6	–	7	0	0	4
29	A	Y	Y	N	N	N	N	Y	N	Y	Y	N	
30	B	T	T	T	T	T	T	T	T	T	T	T	
31	B	F	F	T	F	T	F	F	F	F	F	F	
32	B	T	T	T	F	T	F	T	T	F	F	F	
33	E	2.5	4	3	2.5	0.5	2	2	3	4	2	2	2.5
34	D	3.5	0	3	3	0	2	2	3	3	0	4	2.13
35	A	Y	–	N	Y	N	Y/N	Y	N	Y	–	N	
36	A	Y	–	Y	Y	Y	Y	Y	Y	Y	–	Y	
37	A	Y	–	Y	Y	Y	Y	Y	Y	Y	–	Y	
38	E	4	–	3	4	0	2	2	2	2	–	1	2.22
39	D	6	6	0	0	0	6	0	0	0	0	0	1.64
40	A	N	Y	–	–	–	N	–	N	–	–	–	
41	A	Y	–	–	–	–	Y	–	Y	–	–	–	
42	D	1	0	0	6	1	–	2	1	2	5	0	1.8
43	D	–	0	–	–	3	5	3	1	6	–	0	2.57
44	E	1	4	–	–	–	0	–	1	–	–	–	1.5
45.1	D	6	0	5	4	3	6	2	0	0	5	0	2.82
45.2	E	4	–	4	4	2	2	2	–	–	2	–	2.86
46.1	D	6	0	3	4	3	2	2	2	3	3	5	3
46.2	E	4	–	4	4	2	4	3	4	4	4	–	3.67
47.1	D	–	0	3	1	2	0	2	4	4	3	–	2.11
47.2	E	4	–	3	4	–	2	4	4	4	3	–	3.5
48.1	D	–	0	2	2	2	2	2	4	0	3	0	1.7
48.2	E	4	0	2	2	2	2	4	4	0	–	0	2

Item Scale		A	B	C	D	E	F	G	H	I	J	K	Mean
49.1	D	-	4	-	2	-	2	4	4	0	-	0	2.29
49.2	D	-	-	-	3	-	-	-	2	-	-	-	2.5
50.1	D	4	0	-	3.5	-	4	5	5	0	-	0	2.69
50.2	E	-	-	-	4	2	-	-	4	-	-	-	3.33
51.1	D	6	0	-	3	6	0	-	-	4	-	-	3.17
51.2	E	-	-	-	4	-	3.5	-	-	4	-	-	3.83
52	A	Y	Y	N	Y	Y	N	Y	N	N	N	N	
53	A	Y	N	N	Y	Y	Y	N	N	Y	Y	N	
54	C	2	3	3	4	2	2	3	2	1	3	2	2.45
55	C	2.5	3	3	4	2	4	1	2	2	3	3	2.68
56	C	3	3	4	4	2	4	2	2	4	3	2	3
57	C	3.5	2	3	4	0	2	2	1	2	3	2	2.23
58	A	Y	N	Y	Y	N	Y	Y	N	N	Y	Y	
59	A	Y	Y	N	Y	N	Y	Y	N	N	Y	N	
60	D	7	5	5	6	5	3	5	4	5	6	5	5.09
61	D	7	6	4	7	3	3	4	0	4	4.5	5	4.32
62	D	3	3	4	4	0	3	2	4	3	5	0	2.82
63	D	6	0	0	4	0	2	2	0	5	0	0	1.73
64	D	4	0	3	4	1	-	1	0	0	2	0	1.5
65	D	6	5	7	7	5	5	5	5	0	5	-	5
66	A	Y	Y	Y	Y	Y	-	N	Y	Y	Y	Y	
67	A	Y	Y	Y	N	N	-	Y	Y	-	Y	Y	
68	-	-	-	-	-	-	-	-	-	-	-	-	
69	-	-	-	-	-	-	-	-	-	-	-	-	
70	-	-	-	-	-	-	-	-	-	-	-	-	
71	A	Y	Y	Y	Y	Y	Y	Y	Y	-	N	-	
72	A	Y	Y	Y	Y	Y	Y	Y	Y	Y	N	-	
73	A	Y	Y	Y	Y	Y	Y	Y	Y	Y	N	-	
74	A	Y	Y	N	Y	Y	Y	N	N	Y	N	-	
75	A	N	N	N	Y	Y	Y	N	N	Y	N	N	
76	A	N	Y	N	N	Y	Y	Y	N	Y	N	N	
77	A	Y	Y	N	Y	N	Y	Y	Y	N	N	N	
78	A	Y	Y	N	N	N	N	N	Y	N	N	N	
79	A	Y	Y	N	Y	Y	Y	Y	Y	N	N	Y	
80	A	Y	Y	Y	Y	Y	Y	Y	Y	Y	Y	Y	
81	A	N	N	N	N	N	N	Y	Y	N	N	N	
82	A	N	N	N	N	N	N	Y	Y	Y	N	N	
83	A	Y	N	Y	N	Y	N	N	Y	Y	N	N	
84	A	-	-	-	Y	N	N	Y	-	-	Y	N	
85	A	-	Y	-	N	N	Y	Y	Y	-	Y	N	
86	C	1.5	4	-	-	4	3	2	2	1	3	2	2.5
87	A	Y	Y	-	Y	Y	Y	Y	Y	N	Y	Y	
88	A	Y	-	-	-	N	-	Y	Y	Y	N	N	
89	A	Y	Y	Y	Y	N	Y	N	Y	Y	Y	Y	
90	A	Y	Y	Y	Y	Y	N	Y	Y	Y	Y	Y	
91	A	Y	Y	N	Y	N	N	Y	Y	Y	N	N	
92	F	S	S	N	M	S	S	S	M	S	S	S	
93	A	N	-	N	N	N	N	N	Y	N	N	-	
94	F	S	M	S	M	S	S	S	A	S	M	A	
95	A	Y	Y	Y	Y	N	Y	N	Y	N	N	N	
96	A	N	Y	Y	N	E	Y	N	H	-	N	K	
97	A	Y	N	N	Y	Y	Y	Y	N	N	Y	N	
98	A	N	Y	N	Y	N	N	N	N	N	Y	N	
99	A	Y	Y	Y	Y	Y	Y	N	N	N	Y	N	

Standards to Consider for Version 2 Protocol

In addition to the recommendations in Chapter 8, and the results of the statistical analysis, the following key aspects of good mental health services should be considered for incorporation in Version 2 of the Protocol.

Education

A3.1   Multi-disciplinary clinical audit is a routine part of clinical work. Audits are followed by appropriate action and the outcomes monitored.

A3.2   Guidelines on effective methods of cognitive, behavioural and family therapies, their indications, and applications for both users and carers, are part of routine audit and training in all units responsible for the treatment of people with schizophrenia and SMI.

A3.3   The proportion of health authorities' and other purchasers' budgets devoted to training mental health professionals is at the level of the mean of NHS expenditure under this head. Continuing professional education is mandatory for all grades, continuous from the time of recruitment, and directed towards the maintenance of explicit standards.

A3.4   Initiatives are directed towards explaining the nature of schizophrenia, its impact on those afflicted and on others, with particular attention to misconceptions about the frequency of dangerous and criminal behaviour.

Treatment and care

A3.5   Everyone with SMI is offered a yearly physical examination, including the effects of poverty or self-neglect and any side-effects of medication.

A3.6   Healthcare professionals have the skills needed to supervise and provide the whole range of treatments and care, including physical, cognitive and behavioural therapies, and family, social, occupational and welfare interventions.

A3.7   A full range of settings is available, providing effective environments for the interventions in A3.6.

A3.8   Contracts specify CPN caseloads including: (a) the balance between SMI and less severe disorders, (b) caseload size with reference to local need and casemix, eg 15-20 for teams caring mainly for the SMI, (c) continuing education (e.g. Thorn) and personal development schemes.

A3.9   The number of acute in-patient places is appropriate for the needs of the local population.

Commissioning

A3.10   Service contracts contain explicit statements concerning the availability, from skilled practitioners, of treatments such as clozapine and other medications, cognitive and behaviour therapy, family and social interventions, access to forensic and secure provision, and all components of a rehabilitation service.

A3.11   Purchasers demonstrate that providers, users and carers were consulted during the development of strategic plans. In particular, there is evidence that provider clinicians have been engaged in the development and negotiation of contracts.

A3.12   The financial arrangements and relationships between GPFHs and the specialist mental health service are such that it is advantageous to employ community psychiatric nurses to ensure continuity of care for people with severe long term mental illness.

A3.13   NHS and LA purchasers and providers collaborate in a single plan for close joint working, with clear stages and timetable.

Leadership and morale

A3.14   There is a shared vision between purchaser and provider; commitment to clear aims and achievable targets; shared audit and accountability between managers and professionals; organisational stability.

A3.15   There is strong clinical leadership, with appropriate senior staff levels for the population served, stability of tenure and good administrative back-up.

Methods of measurement

A3.16   The quality, accessibility and distribution of mental health statistics and sociodemographics is of sufficient quality to describe and audit the local services.

A3.17   A clinician-, patient- and manager-friendly register system is in place for routine clinical use including CPA; and also for audit, patient and carer information, commissioning, public health and administrative purposes.

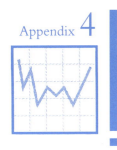

Glossary of Definitions & Descriptions

A&C:	Administrative and Clerical
A&E:	Accident & Emergency
ASW:	Approved Social Worker
C&R:	Control & Restraint
CMHN:	Community Mental Health Nurse
CMHT:	Community Mental Health Team
CPA:	Care Programme Approach
CPN:	Community Psychiatric Nurse
CRU:	College Research Unit
CSAG:	Clinical Standards Advisory Group
CSAG-S:	Clinical Standards Advisory Group – Schizophrenia Study
DGH:	District General Hospital
DHA:	District Health Authority
DMU:	NHS Directly Managed Unit
ECR:	Extra Contractual Referral
FCE:	Finished Consultant Episodes
FHSA:	Family Health Services Authority
GP:	General Practitioner
GPFH:	General Practice Fund Holder
HAS:	Health Advisory Service
HIP:	Health Investment Plan
IT:	Information Technology
LASS:	Local Authority Social Services
MDO:	Mentally disordered offender
MDT:	Multidisciplinary Team
MHA:	Mental Health Act 1983
MHAC:	Mental Health Act Commission
MHS:	Mental Health Service
MIAG:	Mental Illness Action Group
OT:	Occupational Therapy
PAS:	Patient Administration System
RCPsych:	Royal College of Psychiatrists
RSU:	Regional Secure Unit
S117 MHA:	Section 117 of the Mental Health Act 1983
S133 MHA:	Section 133 of the Mental Health Act 1983
S136 MHA:	Section 136 of the Mental Health Act 1983
UPA8:	Underprivileged Areas Score (Jarman indices)
SCZ:	Schizophrenia
SMI:	Severe Mental Illness
SSD:	Social Service Department
SW:	Social Work

Advocacy - the communicating of expressed needs by, or on behalf of, a user to service providers.

Audit - 'The systematic critical analysis of the quality of care, including the procedures used for diagnosis and treatment, the use of resources, and the resulting outcome and quality of life for the patient'. (DOH 1989)

Carer - a relative or friend of a user who is actively involved in their care.

Care Management - From the 1 April 1993 local authority social service departments have become the lead agency responsible for assessing, purchasing and monitoring the community care of people with disabilities linked to mental illness, old age, physical disabilities and learning difficulties. Social Service Inspectorate guidelines identify seven core tasks of care management: publishing information, determining the level of assessment needed, assessing need, care planning, implementing the care plan, monitoring and review. There is considerable flexibility in the way each authority can structure care management. However, authorities are expected to produce community care plans consistent with those of health authorities, and to produce individual care packages in collaboration with medical, nursing and other relevant groups.

Case Management - Similar to care management; assessment and care planning is carried out by a case manager who co-ordinates the delivery of care and is responsible for monitoring and review. A case manager may also act as a key worker.

Clozapine - a recently introduced psychotropic drug still under test currently used to treat treatment-resistant schizophrenia.

Community Mental Health Nurse - see Community Psychiatric Nurse.

CPA: Care Programme Approach - The Care Programme Approach was introduced in the NHS in April 1991. Health Care Providers are required to develop, in collaboration with local social services departments, individual packages of care (care programmes) for all in-patients about to be discharged from hospital and all new patients accepted by the specialist psychiatric services. Care programmes may range from 'minimal' single worker assessment and monitoring, for individuals with less severe mental health and social needs, to complex multidisciplinary assessments and treatment.

CRU: College Research Unit - An independent multidisciplinary research unit attached to the Royal College of Psychiatrists. Commissioned to draft standards and provide research and office support for the CSAG-S schizophrenia study.

CSAG: Clinical Standards Advisory Group - The CSAG was established in 1991 under S62 of the NHS and Community Care Act as an independent source of expert advice to UK Health Ministers and NHS bodies on standards of clinical care for, and on access and availability of services to, NHS patients. The remit to study services for people with schizophrenia (CSAG-S) was set in August 1993.

DMU: Directly Managed Unit (NHS) - A hospital or community provider service which has not yet sought or achieved Trust status. DMUs remain under the management of DHAs, although in other respects, the "purchaser-provider" separation is identical to Trusts.

FCE: Finished Consultant Episodes - The point at which a patient is referred back to the care of a GP or other specialist service and a discharge report completed.

GPFH: General Practice Fund Holder - GP practices with lists above a certain size are free to apply for their own NHS budget to obtain a defined range of services. Budgets also cover practice staff costs, improvement to premises and drug costs.

Keyworker - An identified person who has a defined responsibility towards a specific user of services, usually with some responsibility for service provision and monitoring of care.

Outreach - Services which rely primarily on home visiting and in vivo interventions.

Perverse Incentives - Contractual agreements which may encourage service providers to adopt practices or policies which run counter to good clinical management e.g. extra funding for increased length of in-patient stay, the use of episode based monitoring (FCEs) as a contract currency.

S117 MHA: Section 117 of the Mental Health Act 1983 - Section 117 applies to individuals detained under Section 3, 37, 47 or 48 who cease to be detained and are discharged from hospital. It is the responsibility of the RMO to ensure a keyworker is nominated and provides after-care services, in conjunction with Local Authority Social Services, until they are satisfied that the individual no longer needs such care.

S133 MHA: Section 133 of the Mental Health Act 1983 - Section 133 places a duty on managers of hospitals to inform nearest relatives of the discharge of detained patients where practicable, unless the patient or relative has requested otherwise.

S136 MHA: Section 136 of the Mental Health Act 1983 - A police officer can detain a person in a public place who appears to be "suffering from mental disorder" and is in "immediate need of care or control", and remove them to 'a place of safety'.

UPA8: Underprivileged Areas Score (Jarman indices) - The UPA8 is based on eight census indices, being the percentage of people in the local population with the following characteristics; people aged 65+, children aged <4, social class 5, unemployed, single-parent households, overcrowding, highly mobile people and ethnic minorities. Each item is weighted according to GP's views of how much they think it contributes to their workload. The weighted sum, standardised and normalised, constitutes the "Jarman score"; the score can be used as an indicator of deprivation in a geographically defined population and as an approximate indicator of morbidity.

Special Hospital - Hospitals for psychiatric patients who require care in conditions of special security. In England 3 hospitals are managed by the Special Hospitals Services Authority; Broadmoor, Rampton and Ashworth. In Scotland there is a State Hospital at Carstairs Junction.

Supervision Register - From 1 April 1994 all Purchasers and Providers of Mental Health Services are required to have in place a register which ensures the identification and registration of all severely mentally ill people at risk of causing serious harm to themselves or others or of serious neglect.

User - a person with a mental health problem who is receiving mental health care services.

Members of the CSAG Schizophrenia Committee

Members of the CSAG Schizophrenia Committee

Chairman: Professor Andrew Sims MA MD FRCPsych FRCP Ed
Professor of Psychiatry, University of Leeds.

Dr. Charles Brooker PhD MSc BA RMN RNT DipNEd
Director of Nursing Research, SCHAAR, University of Sheffield.

Professor Kevin Gournay MPhil PhD C Psychol AFBPsS RN
Professor of Mental Health, Middlesex University.

Mr David Joannides BA CQSW
Deputy Director of Social Services, Dorset County Council.

Ms Jennifer Hunt MPhil BA RGN FRCN
Director, Nursing Research Initiative for Scotland. Previously Nursing Practice Consultant.

Dr. Robin Graeme McCreadie DSc MD FRCPsych DPM
Consultant Psychiatrist, Crichton Royal Hospital.

Dr. Nuala Sterling CBE MB FRCP
Consultant Physician Geriatric Medicine, Southampton University Hospitals Trust.

Dr. Hilary Stirland MB BS FFPHM D(Obst)RCOG
Director of Public Health, Merton Sutton & Wandsworth Health Authority.

Dr. Colin Waine OBE FRCGP FRCPath
Director of Primary Care, Sunderland Health Commission.

Dr Richard Williams MB,ChB FRCPsych DPM MHSM
Director of the NHS Health Advisory Service, Consultant Child and Adolescent Psychiatrist, United Bristol Healthcare NHS Trust.

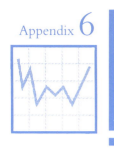

Members of the Research and Visiting Teams

Research Team – College Research Unit, The Royal College of Psychiatrists

Professor John Wing CBE MD PhD FRCPsych	Director
Susannah Rix BSc	Research Psychologist
Roy Curtis MA DipClinPsychol MBA	Senior Research Fellow
Alan Beadsmoore MA BA RMN	Senior Research Worker (Jan-Sept 1994)

Members of The Visiting Teams

Mr Ian Baguley RMN CPN Cert
Clinical Nurse Specialist, Kings Fund Project Worker, Tameside Community Priority Services Trust.

Mr Allan Brown MSc CQSW
Principal Officer (Mental Health), Dorset Social Services.

Dr. T.S. Brugha MD MRCPsych
Senior Lecturer and Consultant Psychiatrist, Leicester.

Professor Tom Burns MD FRCPsych
Professor of Community Psychiatry, St. Georges Hospital, London.

Dr. Michael Doherty MRCPsych
Consultant Psychiatrist, Belfast City Hospital, Health and Social Services Trust, Northern Ireland.

Dr. Richard A. Gater MB,ChB MRCPsych MSc
Senior Lecturer in Psychiatry, University of Manchester, Honorary Consultant Psychiatrist, South Manchester, University Hospitals NHS Trust.

Professor Glynn Harrison MD MRCPsych
Academic Dept. Psychiatry, Happerley Hospital, Nottingham.

Mr Edward McLaughlin RMN
Senior Nurse Manager, Oxfordshire Mental Health Care, NHS Trust.

Dr. Lesley Parkinson BSc MSc PGC Health Econ.
Chief Clinical Psychologist, Riverside Mental Health Trust.

Mr Dean Repper RMN MSc
Quality Advisor, Nottingham Health Care, NHS Trust.

Ms Sarah Robson SRN RMN CIM

Senior Charge Nurse, Hellesdon Hospital, Norwich.

Ms Jean Spencer Dip Cot SROT

Team Leader, Community Support Team North, Southwark.

Ms Rosemary Telford BA MSc MAppSci

Consultant Psychologist, Community Health Sheffield, NHS Trust.

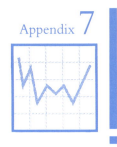

Mental Health Policy Developments 1957 – 1994

1957	Report of the Royal Commission on the Law relating to mental Illness and Deficiency
1959	Mental Health Act
1962	Hospital Plan for England and Wales, Ministry of Health White Paper
1975	Better Services for the Mentally Ill. DHSS White Paper
1976	Joint Care Planning: Health and Local Authorities. DHSS Circular
1981	Care in Action. A Handbook of Policies and Priorities for the Health and Personal Social Services in England. DHSS
1983	Mental Health Act
	Care in the Community. DHSS Consultative Document
1985	Community Care with special reference to adult mentally ill and mentally handicapped people. House of Commons Social Services Committee Report
1986	Making a Reality of Community Care. Audit Commission
1988	Community Care: Agenda for Action. Sir Roy Griffiths
	The Report of the Committee of Inquiry into the Care and After-Care of Sharon Camphell
1989	Caring for People: Community Care in the Next Decade and Beyond. White Paper
1990	NHS and Community Care Act
	Community Care. House of Commons Social Services Committee Report.
1991	Care Programme Approach
	Mental Illness Specific Grant
1992	Mental Illness a Key Area in "Health of the Nation". White Paper
	Joint DH/Home Office Review of Services for Mentally Disordered Offenders [Chair: J Reed]
1993	Mental Illness Key Area Handbook
	Mental Health Task Force set up.
	Review of Legal Powers on the Care of Mentally Ill People in the Community
	Secretary of State for Health's 10 point plan (see below)
1994	Introducing supervision registers from 1st April 1994. DH guidance.
	Discharge of mentally disordered people and their continuing care in the community. DH guidance.
	Mental Health Nursing Review. DH
	The care of Christopher Clunis. [Chair: J Ritchie]
	Better off in the Community? The Care of People who are Seriously Mentally Ill. House of Commons Health Committee Report
	Finding a Place. Audit Commission
	Mental Illness Key Area Handbook (2nd Edition)
1995	Mental Health (Patients in the Community) Bill

Secretary of State's Ten Point Plan
(Press Release H93/908 of 12 August 1993)

Plan for developing safe and successful community care

1   Review by the Clinical Standards Advisory Group of standards of care for people with schizophrenia.

2   Agreed work programme for the Mental Health Task Force.

3   Ensure Health Authority and GP fund-holder plans cover the essential needs for mental health services.

4   The London Implementation Group to take forward an action plan to improve mental health services in the capital.

5   Better training for keyworkers under the Care Programme Approach.

6   Publication of the Review of Legal Powers.

7   Seek legislation for
    a) the new power of supervised discharge
    b) extending leave under Section 3 to 1 year.

8   Publication of the revised Code of Practice for MHA.

9   Guidance on discharge of mentally disordered people.

10 Development of better information systems.

Government Response to CSAG's Report on Schizophrenia

Services for people with a mental illness

Government strategy

1. For almost twenty years it has been accepted policy that people with a mental illness are best cared for through a comprehensive range of locally based health and social services, including suitable housing and opportunities for employment where appropriate, rather than in large, remote institutions.

2. Health and local authorities need to arrange for a broad spectrum of care including, for example, provision in a domestic setting by the statutory and independent sector agencies, staffed residential accommodation and provision for sufficient, good quality in-patient care for those who cannot cope in the community.

3. The key issue is that no one agency can provide the range and type of services required. They must work together to provide modern methods of treatment and social support giving value for money in the most appropriate setting.

4. Health and social services for people with a mental illness need to be developed in the context of the Health of the Nation Initiative where mental illness is one of the 5 key areas and within the general framework of responsibilities set out in relation to Care in the Community. The inclusion of mental illness as a key area means that improving the health and social functioning of mentally ill people is a Government priority.

5. The focus of attention for both health and local authorities is now on the provision of services for severely mentally ill people so as to ensure they do not fall through the net of care. Severely mentally ill people need a variety of services and support if they are to be maintained in the community and in August 1993 Mrs Bottomley, Secretary of State for Health, launched a Ten Point Plan to reinforce care in the community for this group.

6. The Ten Point Plan is being implemented in conjunction with other initiatives and includes:-

- Introduction of the Mental Health (Patients in the Community) Bill to provide more effective care and supervision by way of a new power of supervised discharge";

- Publication of a revised Code of Practice on the Mental Health Act 1983;

- The issue of guidance on hospital discharge in May 1994;

- Circular LAC(94)6 of February 1994 to local authorities on the Mental Illness Specific Grant (MISG) advising them that projects funded by the grant must be targeted on those most at risk;

- The introduction of supervision registers from April 1994 as part of the Care Programme Approach;

- Publication of the Mental Health Task Force reports on Mental Health in London;

- Publication of a 2nd edition of the Mental Illness Key Area Handbook for Health and Local Authorities;

- Preparation of a Guide to the Arrangements for Inter-Agency Co-operation for the Protection of Severely Mentally Ill People; and

- Circular LAC(95)4 of February 1995 to local authorities on the MISG distributing an extra £10 million for 1995/96 to target services and resources even more sharply on severely mentally ill people.

CSAG Recommendations

The following paragraphs reproduce CSAG's recommendations from Chapter 8 of the Report - in italics - followed by the Government's Response to each recommendation.

1.   The Version 2 protocol should be developed through wider use by clinicians, managers and commissioners as part of their local audit measures.

The CSAG Protocol forms a good basis for purchasers and providers to assess the level and quality of services provided for severely mentally ill people with schizophrenia as part of their local audit procedures. We would wish to encourage its' use as part of a programme to develop services and raise standards.

2.   Commissioners should, after consulting users and carers, agree with service providers' explicit statements of the standards to be achieved locally and consider referring in these statements to use of the Version 2 protocol, as developed, as one of the methods of auditing clinical and managerial aspects of the district service.

It is important that standards of care for schizophrenia are made explicit so that the relevant professionals, users and carers, as well as managers, know what the aims of the service are and how they measure up to those standards. Use and development of the Protocol can help to set the appropriate local standards.

3.   The NHS Executive should, where it has serious concerns about standards and the effectiveness of local audit to identify weaknesses, consider using the Version 2 protocol itself or inviting an independent agency to investigate in more detail.

The Protocol can be used as a tool to raise standards via local audit and the NHS performance management system. Outside agencies can be brought in where it is appropriate to use their specialised skills and knowledge.

*4.	The place of skilled diagnosis within the clinical and social assessment of people with severe mental illness in indicating priority for services should be recognised in contracts, supported and audited.*

Skilled diagnosis is a key element in recognising the most effective treatment required for severely mentally ill people and this should be seen as part of the need to ensure the provision of an appropriate range of trained professionals to look after this vulnerable group.

*5.	A simple register system should be developed to support the information requirements of the Care Programme Approach, with Supervision Registers and Supervised Discharge as subsets, and to underpin clinical work with high priority groups and clinical audit.*

This recommendation is fully in line with our Health of the Nation strategy to improve the co-ordination of care of severely mentally ill people. However, registers need to be simple to operate and understand, provide effective support to health and social care professionals in arranging suitable packages of care and at the same time, not be a bureaucratic burden on authorities. We are developing detailed proposals for the introduction of comprehensive systems, including the supervision registers which are already in place.

*6.	The principles of multi-disciplinary and multi-professional audit should be applied in all agencies providing care for designated groups such as the severely mentally ill. This will require harmonisation of methods of data collection by local mental health teams, general practices and social services.*

No one agency has all the skills, expertise, knowledge or services to provide an effective range of care for severely mentally ill people. There is a clear need to adopt a multi-disciplinary and multi-professional approach for this vulnerable group to include audit and information gathering systems wherever practicable. We have issued a draft Guide to Inter-Agency working for the care and protection of severely mentally ill people which is being revised in the light of responses to the consultation exercise.

*7.	CSAG should repeat its district surveys, following discussion with districts of the visiting teams' assessments of standards and priorities for change.*

The CSAG protocol can now be taken forward by the NHS as part of the overall local performance management and quality system control to ensure standards are monitored properly.

Printed in the United Kingdom for HMSO
Dd 0301198 C140 8/95 65536 328978 28/33217